Management of Infertility for the MRCOG and Beyond

Published titles in the MRCOG and Beyond series

Neonatology for the MRCOG *by Peter Dear and Simon Newell*

Menstrual Problems for the MRCOG *by Mary Ann Lumsden, Jane Norman and Hilary Critchley*

Gynaecological and Obstetric Pathology for the MRCOG *by Harold Fox and C. Hilary Buckley, with a chapter on Cervical Cytology by Dulcie V. Coleman*

Forthcoming titles in the series

Antenatal Disorders

Early Pregnancy Issues

Fetal Medicine

Gynaecological Oncology

Gynaecological Urology

Intrapartum Care

Management of Infertility

Molecular Medicine

Paediatric and Adolescent Gynaecology

Reproductive Endocrinology

Management of Infertility for the MRCOG and Beyond

Allan Templeton
Premila W Ashok
Siladitya Bhattacharya
M Rafet Gazvani
Mark Hamilton
Susan Macmillan
Ashalatha Shetty

Series Editor: Peter Milton

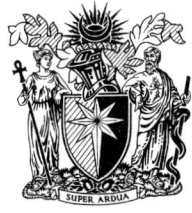

RCOG Press

First published 2000

Reprinted 2003

© Royal College of Obstetricians and Gynaecologists 2000

ISBN 1–900364–29-8

Published by the **RCOG Press** at the
Royal College of Obstetricians and Gynaecologists
27 Sussex Place, Regent's Park
London NW1 4RG

Registered charity No. 213280

Cover illustration:
RCOG Editor: Jane Moody

Typesetting: Saxon Graphics Limited, Derby, UK
Printing: J W Arrowsmith Limited, Winterstoke Road, Bristol BS3 2NT

Contents

About the authors

Premila W. Ashok MBBS MRCOG MFFP
Specialist Registrar, Assisted Reproduction Unit, Aberdeen Maternity Hospital, Cornhill Road, Aberdeen AB25 2ZD

Siladitya Bhattacharya MD MRCOG
Senior Lecturer, Department of Obstetrics and Gynaecology, Aberdeen Maternity Hospital, Cornhill Road, Aberdeen AB25 2ZD

M. Rafet Gazvani MRCOG
Clinical Lecturer, Department of Obstetrics and Gynaecology, Aberdeen Maternity Hospital, Cornhill Road, Aberdeen AB25 2ZD

Mark Hamilton MD FRCOG
Honorary Senior Lecturer, Assisted Reproduction Unit, Aberdeen Maternity Hospital, Cornhill Road, Aberdeen AB25 2ZD

Susan Macmillan MRCOG
Clinical Research Fellow, Department of Obstetrics and Gynaecology, Aberdeen Maternity Hospital, Cornhill Road, Aberdeen AB25 2ZD

Ashalatha Shetty DGO MRCOG MRCP II (Ireland)
Clinical Research Fellow, Assisted Reproduction Unit, Aberdeen Maternity Hospital, Cornhill Road, Aberdeen AB25 2ZD

Allan Templeton MD FRCOG
Professor of Obstetrics and Gynaecology, University of Aberdeen, Aberdeen Maternity Hospital, Cornhill Road, Aberdeen AB25 2ZD

Series Editor: Peter Milton MD FRCOG
Consultant Obstetrician and Gynaecologist, Addenbrooke's and Rosie Maternity Hospital, Robinson Way, Cambridge CB2 2SW

Preface

Infertility affects one in seven couples in the Western world and this figure may rise as more women are delaying parenthood. It is a major cause of psychological and marital stress and, hence, deserves to be managed as a disease entity along with more traditionally recognised diseases. There are wide variations in infertility services throughout the UK and in some cases dissatisfaction with provision, in particular regarding counselling and the access to assisted conception. Although the initial management of the infertile couple can be carried out in primary care, more complex management should take place in a dedicated infertility clinic where treatment using evidence-based guidelines can be instituted.

Every MRCOG candidate must have a broad knowledge of infertility management and this volume, which has been written jointly by members of one of the most prestigious infertility clinics in the UK, provides the data upon which this knowledge can be developed. It will also prove, I am sure, to be extremely popular with specialists in established practice seeking to update their knowledge of this important aspect of gynaecological practice. The book is sure to be an extremely popular addition to the 'MRCOG and Beyond' series.

Peter Milton
January 2000

1 The management of infertility

Introduction

Infertility affects one in seven couples in industrialised countries. There has been no major change in prevalence in recent years, but more couples are seeking help than previously. This is associated with a greater awareness of the problem and also the availability of more effective treatment, particularly *in vitro* fertilisation (IVF). There are, however, wide variations in clinical practice, and patient dissatisfaction with services continues to be highlighted.

Infertility can cause considerable psychological distress to couples. The United Nations states that reproductive health is 'a state of complete physical, mental and social well-being and not merely the absence of disease or infirmity in all matters relating to the reproductive system and to its function and processes'. Infertility should therefore be considered a disease worthy of investigation and treatment (RCOG 1998a).

Definitions of infertility vary considerably, particularly in relation to the duration of regular unprotected intercourse. Circumstances will differ but couples should be considered individually and seen whenever *they* think there is a problem. Often there are factors such as the woman's age, previous surgery or irregular periods that warrant investigation earlier than the usual one or two years of trying. Generally, couples appreciate a service that provides rapid and efficient diagnosis, frank discussion of prognosis, and a clearly agreed plan of management. Two major issues have shaped the provision of infertility services in recent years:

- the introduction of an evidence-based approach to management and, in particular, treatment
- the availability of assisted reproduction.

One of the major problems in the current provision of services is limited access to IVF and related techniques.

Epidemiology

Despite differences in approach and definition, most studies indicate that approximately 15% of all couples will experience difficulties in conceiving (Table 1.1). Of these, about one-half will be subfertile rather than infertile and will eventually go on to conceive, either spontaneously or with the help of simple advice and remedies. The other half will remain infertile and will require more sophisticated treatment, of the kind usually only available in established infertility clinics. In all, approximately half will have primary infertility and the other half will have secondary infertility. Current information also suggests a much higher incidence of miscarriage and ectopic pregnancy among subfertile women.

DEFINITION OF INFERTILITY

Primary infertility   Couples will never have conceived at any stage

Secondary infertility   Couples will have had a pregnancy although not necessarily a successful one

---

A number of studies now indicate that the likelihood of a spontaneous pregnancy occurring in a subfertile woman is greatly influenced by her age, the duration of infertility and the occurrence of a previous pregnancy. This is so for all categories of infertility, but especially for unexplained infertility, and this is further addressed in Chapter 7. These issues are clearly important for clinical management, and also for assessing the outcome of new interventions and treatment. The woman's characteristics can also have a major effect on the likelihood of any treatment being successful.

KEY POINTS
- Approximately 15% of all couples will experience difficulties in conceiving.
- A young woman with a short duration of infertility and a previous pregnancy is much more likely to become pregnant spontaneously than an older woman with a longer duration of infertility and no pregnancies.

Table 1.1 Prevalence of infertility	
Couples who will experience infertility	15%
Couples whose infertility remains unresolved	8%
Those with primary infertility	4%
Those with secondary infertility	4%

Aetiology

In this book aetiology will be addressed in the context of the management of the individual clinical problems. Generally speaking causal factors can be associated with:

- lifestyle (e.g. weight and smoking)
- genetic causes (e.g. sex chromosome anomalies and Kallman syndrome)
- acquired causes (e.g. following injury and infection).

LIFESTYLE

Smoking, both male and female, has been associated with subfertility as well as poorer treatment outcomes. Although the association is quite strong, a causal relationship is still to be clearly established. It is important to determine, when taking the history, whether there are any other lifestyle factors that may be contributory.

GENETIC CAUSES

The clinical presentation will usually provoke appropriate investigations in relation to genetic causes, but there are now additional concerns about the implications for the offspring. Using assisted reproduction techniques, the infertility of this generation can often be overcome, but the problem may be handed on to the next generation.

ACQUIRED CAUSES

In relation to acquired problems, two stand out in the female:

- the consequences of surgery on the reproductive tract
- infection of the upper tract, particularly when caused by *Chlamydia trachomatis*.

The association between chlamydia and tubal infertility is now well established. It is accepted that chlamydia is the major preventable cause of tubal disease in the western world. It may turn out to be the major preventable cause of infertility when its effect on the male is also considered.

KEYPOINTS
- Smoking has been associated with subfertility as well as poorer treatment outcomes.
- Genetic problems may be passed on to the next generation.
- Chlamydia may be the major preventable cause of infertility.

Diagnostic categories

Couples are usually managed in the context of the major diagnostic category to which they have been assigned. These categories are based not so much on diagnosis, but on functional and pragmatic considerations which facilitate treatment (Table 1.2). However, not all couples will fit neatly into one category and several problems may have to be managed simultaneously, such as inducing ovulation in an anovulatory woman in order to carry out donor insemination.

The distribution of couples in each of the diagnostic categories will vary from clinic to clinic depending on referral patterns: typical figures are shown. Couples with primary infertility are more frequent in all of the categories except tubal, where secondary infertility is more frequent. This highlights the fact that pregnancy is a risk factor for the development of tubal disease, presumably associated with opportunities for ascending infection, whether after early or late pregnancy. Table 1.2 highlights the importance of investigating the male partner in cases of secondary infertility, even where he has been responsible for a recent pregnancy.

Table 1.2 Diagnostic categories and distribution of couples with primary and secondary infertility

Diagnostic category	Primary (%)	Secondary (%)
Male	25	20
Ovulation	20	15
Tubal	15	40
Endometriosis	10	5
Unexplained	30	20

Prevention of infertility

Unfortunately the opportunities for the prevention of infertility appear to be limited. However, there is now much more awareness of the importance of appropriate surgical techniques when operating on young women whose fertility may be an issue. Similarly, the prevention of chlamydial infection is receiving much more attention and gynaecologists need to be much more aware of the risks of ascending infection in women. Recently, highly sensitive nucleic acid-based tests have been developed to detect chlamydia and these can be carried out in first void urine samples or vulval swabs, as well as cervical swabs. Any woman at risk, and this particularly applies to women under the age of 25 years, who are having uterine instrumentation for any reason, should be tested for chlamydia.

Eventually reductions in the prevalence of chlamydia will result from better public awareness as well as population-based screening.

KEYPOINT
- Any woman at risk who is having uterine instrumentation for any reason should be tested for the presence of *Chlamydia trachomatis*.

Effective treatments

In recent years a much more critical approach to the effective management of the infertile couple has emerged. This is partly associated with the introduction and increasing use of evidence-based medicine. Evaluation of the literature in a systematic way has demonstrated that many of the treatments previously used in the management of the infertile couple were ineffective and should no longer be used. Areas where the evidence does not support treatment include:

- drug treatment of the male
- drug treatment for infertility-related endometriosis
- (probably) the use of clomiphene for unexplained infertility.

Where there is continuing uncertainty, a treatment should only be used within the context of randomised clinical trials.

At the same time there has been increasing dependence on more complex treatments, including ovarian stimulation and intrauterine insemination and, particularly, *in vitro* fertilisation (IVF) and related techniques. These techniques are not effective in all circumstances, having as they do a relatively low success rate per cycle of intervention.

As previously noted, it is now well established that a number of patient characteristics have enormous importance in predicting the likelihood of a spontaneous pregnancy, whatever the clinical diagnosis. A young woman with a short duration of infertility and a previous pregnancy has a high likelihood of achieving a further spontaneous pregnancy (that is, without treatment or intervention) and it would be very difficult for any of the interventions at our disposal to match this likelihood. It may therefore be appropriate to postpone treatment in these circumstances in the expectation that a pregnancy will occur naturally. The strength of these factors has been quantified in a number of studies, and the results from one such study carried out in Canada are shown in Table 1.3.

Unfortunately, these factors are also the main determinants in assessing the outcome of any intervention. Thus, a young woman in her twenties might expect a greater than 30% chance of a live birth following IVF whereas a woman in her early forties would expect a less than 5% chance (Templeton *et al.* 1996).

COST EFFECTIVENESS

Assessing cost effectiveness is a much more difficult issue. Comparing two similar treatments, one using an expensive drug and the other using a cheap drug, may be easy, particularly if they both have similar pregnancy rates. However, the cheaper drug may be administered over several cycles and produce as good a pregnancy rate as the more expensive drug given for one cycle, but with fewer adverse effects and complications. The issue of cost effectiveness then becomes much more difficult; particularly where there is a risk of multiple pregnancy and associated perinatal morbidity. Nonetheless, the importance of assessing cost and benefits, particularly within the context of randomised studies, is now acknowledged when assessing the overall effects of infertility management.

Table 1.3   Patient characteristics and the likelihood of a live birth (data from Collins *et al.* 1995)

	Factor	(Confidence limits)
Secondary infertility	1.8	(1.2–2.7)
Less than three years infertility	1.7	(1.1–2.5)
Female less than 30 years	1.5	(1.1–2.2)

Unwanted effects of treatment

Three unwanted effects of treatment are highlighted. These are:

- the emotional consequences
- multiple births
- the cancer risk.

EMOTIONAL CONSEQUENCES

The inevitable emotional consequences of infertility can be diminished by a number of important measures. These include the adequate provision of information, better access to services, and more awareness among professionals of the psychological and emotional impact of infertility. Similarly, co-ordination of investigations between the different levels of service and more support when giving the results of tests, particularly if the news is not good, can all help to diminish the problem. The issues that cause most distress to patients are insensitive staff, poor co-ordination of services, inadequate standards of treatment, lack of information, and lack of support when most needed (Table 1.4). Although there is no direct evidence that counselling improves the outcome of fertility treatment, there is good evidence that counselling reduces distress and there is some evidence that distress may affect the outcome of treatment.

Table 1.4 Ranking of patients' views about infertility management (data from Souter et al. 1998)

- The information and explanation given (including written information)
- The doctor's attitude (listening and supportive)
- The way investigations are done (quickly and efficiently)
- Help with emotional side (counselling)
- Waiting time at clinic (and more frequent appointments)

MULTIPLE BIRTH

The high rate of multiple births resulting from infertility treatment remains a major concern. The medical, social and financial consequences are considerable, chiefly because of the excessive morbidity among the survivors of high order multiple births (triplets or more). The problems arise mainly from ovulation induction and IVF treatment. In ovulation induction multiple pregnancies are associated with the difficulties in monitoring follicular development. The recent RCOG evidence-based clinical guideline (1998a) recommends that:

- all centres should adopt protocols, which minimise the risk of multiple pregnancy and ovarian hyperstimulation
- all patients undergoing ovulation induction should be given information about the risks of multiple pregnancy, ovarian hyperstimulation and the possibility of fetal reduction
- ovulation induction with gonadotrophins should only be performed in circumstances which permit daily monitoring of ovarian response (in practice this means daily access to ultrasound monitoring)
- clinics should clearly define the criteria for abandoning cycles and should be prepared to abandon cycles where there is any risk of multiple follicular development.

With IVF the problem relates to the large number of embryos transferred in treatment cycles. Although there is a limit in the UK of three embryos in any cycle, there is increasing evidence that two embryos will suffice in most situations, and all that is achieved when three are transferred is an increase in the rate of multiple pregnancy. It has to be recognised that clinicians and couples feel under considerable pressure to maximise pregnancy rates, but there is an increasing view that multiple gestation is an unacceptable consequence of these pressures.

RISK OF CANCER

There has been increasing concern in recent years about a possible link between drugs given for infertility treatment and the subsequent risk of cancer, particularly ovarian cancer. It is well established that nulliparous women and particularly infertile women are at greater risk of developing ovarian cancer than parous women, but the effects of treatment are less clear. Recent studies should reassure us that any additional effect of drug treatment, if present, is likely to be small, and does not affect women who conceive with such treatment. Nevertheless, the association between ovarian cancer risk and gonadotrophins or prolonged clomiphene use remains uncertain and all patients should be counselled about the putative risks of ovarian cancer associated with ovarian induction therapy.

There is also a responsibility on practitioners to limit the use of gonadotrophins to the lowest effective dose and duration of use (Duckitt and Templeton 1998).

KEYPOINTS
- Services could be improved for infertile couples by providing more help with the emotional aspects of infertility and greater continuity of care.
- All centres should adopt protocols which minimise the risk of multiple pregnancy and ovarian hyperstimulation.
- All patients should be counselled about the putative risks of ovarian cancer associated with ovulation induction therapy.

Context of care

Recent RCOG evidence-based clinical guidelines (1998b) indicate that much of the initial investigation and management of the infertile couple can be carried out in primary care. It is important, however, that there are agreed protocols, based on national guidelines, for investigation and referral. Inevitably the resources and facilities available in secondary care will vary considerably and these will depend on the local circumstances and the population served. Whatever the situation, a basic minimum set of requirements is envisaged:

- The couple should always be managed as a couple.
- Their management should always be discussed in the context of their particular clinical situation and where necessary supported by appropriate written information.
- Patients should be fully involved in decisions regarding their treatment.
- Patients should have access to expert advice and counselling to help them in making their choices and in managing their infertility.
- Secondary care should take place in a dedicated infertility clinic in which there are appropriate facilities and access to trained staff, including doctors, nurses and counsellors.

The guidelines anticipate that these issues should be addressed by all of those involved in the provision of infertility care, including not just the practitioners, but also the patients and the commissioning services. Access to tertiary care, particularly IVF, is limited within the National Health Service in the UK, but it is important that patients should have access to the highest available standards and quality of care, wherever they present.

Conclusion

The two aspects of care which are ranked most highly by patients are the information and explanation given and the doctor's attitude. Many patients also indicate that they would like more written information. Many feel that they are leaving clinics with unresolved questions and without a clear plan of future management. Similarly, prolonged investigation has been a frequent source of frustration and difficulty to many couples. The use of protocols which minimise unnecessary investigations and prevent duplication of tests should facilitate the process of management as well as referral to secondary and tertiary care.

References

Collins, J.A., Burrows, E.A. and Wilan, A.R. (1995) The prognosis for live birth among untreated infertile couples. *Fertil Steril* **64**, 22–8

Duckitt, K. and Templeton, A.A. (1998) Cancer in women with infertility. *Curr Opin Obstet Gynecol* **10**, 199–203

RCOG (1998a) *The Management of Infertility in Secondary Care.* London: RCOG Press (Evidence-based Clinical Guidelines No. 3) pp. 1–8

RCOG (1998b) *The Initial Investigation and Management of the Infertile Couple.* London: RCOG Press (Evidence-based Clinical Guidelines No. 2) pp. 1–11

Souter, V.L., Penney, G., Hopton, J.L. and Templeton, A.A. (1998) Patient satisfaction with the management of infertility. *Hum Reprod* **13**, 1831–6

Templeton, A., Morris, J.K. and Parslow, W. (1996) Factors that affect outcome of *in vitro* fertilisation treatment. *Lancet* **348**, 1402–6

2 The initial assessment of the infertile couple

Introduction

The investigation and management of infertility is a large public health problem and it is essential that the limited resources available are used prudently. The importance of the initial assessment of the infertile couple cannot therefore be overestimated. Individual health authorities can only achieve this through the development of efficient mechanisms for referral and investigation. Adoption of region-wide protocols of basic investigation such as those recently recommended by the Royal College of Obstetricians and Gynaecologists (1998a,b) will be a valuable asset for those involved in the planning of services, founded upon good liaison between medical and nursing staff in both primary and secondary care. Adherence to such protocols facilitates appropriate and timely investigation along standardised paths. This minimises the risks of delay and repetition of tests which couples find particularly demoralising.

Pragmatic definition of infertility

In counselling couples experiencing difficulty in achieving pregnancy, account must be taken of what is a realistic expectation of fertility in normal circumstances. Sound epidemiological data would suggest that conception should occur in 75% of women within 12 months of ceasing contraception and in 90% by two years (Vessey *et al*. 1978). Thus, many would suggest that infertility should be defined as failure to conceive after at least two years of unprotected intercourse. While this may be based on sound epidemiological principles, there may be particular pressures which, in individual cases, lead to couples seeking advice before two years have elapsed.

PRIMARY CARE

The role of the general practitioner is crucial (Hamilton 1992). Infertility represents a deeply personal problem and many individuals will prefer to discuss intimate matters with someone they know and trust. The support that the GP can provide in terms of counselling and preliminary investigations is an excellent foundation for provision of care. Once referral is made to a specialist clinic the stresses imposed on couples may increase, with demands on their time for attendance, the indignity of some of the investigations carried out and the invasion of privacy that occurs. Since it is well recognised that infertility investigation and treatment pose real threats to domestic stability, it is the GP, through knowledge of the couple and their families, who may be in the best position to provide support for those at greatest risk.

All patients should be seen as couples in appropriate surroundings. Facilities should be available to permit examination of both partners and with sufficient time, usually half an hour, set aside to make an adequate overall assessment of the problem.

HOSPITAL CARE

This should be provided in a setting under the clinical direction of a consultant gynaecologist with a special interest in infertility. Patients should be seen in a dedicated infertility clinic with appropriate appointment times to permit thorough evaluation. A team system should be established involving medical, nursing, laboratory (endocrine and semenology) and counselling personnel to facilitate a consistent and co-ordinated approach to care. The level of treatment options available will depend on the expertise of, and the facilities available to, staff at each centre.

KEYPOINTS
- Infertility is defined as failure to conceive after at least two years of unprotected intercourse.
- All patients should be seen as couples in appropriate surroundings.
- A team system should be established to facilitate a consistent and co-ordinated approach to care.

The infertility consultation

Any couple worried about their fertility should be seen by their GP, regardless of the duration of their infertility. It is unusual for couples to present if this is less than a year. In these circumstances, unless there is a clear indication on the basis of history or examination of either partner, further investigation is usually unnecessary. Merely providing the couple with an outline of their excellent potential fertility over the next year may be all that is required to set their minds at rest. However, couples who present early may themselves have particular concerns or be aware of a problem which merits sympathetic discussion. A little more urgency may be required in the investigation of couples where the female partner is over 35 years of age.

Steps in the process of investigation of infertility should be discussed at the outset with the couple in the expectation that all necessary tests would be complete within four months. The sequence with which tests are performed is, to some extent, standardised for all but may vary if history or examination findings suggest otherwise. Initial investigations are inexpensive, non-invasive and likely to yield useful information.

Points requiring particular attention in the history and examination of the couple are shown in Table 2.1. A psychological assessment of the impact of perceived infertility on individual and couple would also be required.

KEYPOINTS

- The success rate for the treatment of infertility declines with increasing duration of infertility and increasing age.
- All necessary tests should be completed within four months; these are inexpensive, noninvasive and likely to yield useful information.
- A genital examination should be performed even without a positive finding in the history. A small proportion of men will exhibit unsuspected genital pathology, which may have an important bearing on their health in general, and not just their infertility.
- Adnexal pathology such as endometriosis should be borne in mind, particularly for those with a suggestive history.

Table 2.1 World Health Organization values for 'normal' semen analysis

Volume	2–5 ml
Liquefaction time	Within 30 minutes
Concentration	> 20 M/ml
Motility	> 50% progressive motility
Morphology	> 30% normal forms
White blood cells	< I M/ml

Investigation of infertility
History

MALE

Infertility: Previous evidence of fertility, and if so with present partner or not

Duration of infertility and time to achieve previous pregnancies, if any

Previous investigation and treatment

Medical: History of:

- sexually transmitted disease
- epididymitis
- mumps orchitis
- testicular maldescent

- chronic disease
- drug/alcohol abuse
- recent febrile illness
- recurrent urinary tract infection

Surgical:

Herniorrhaphy — Torsion

Testicular injury — Orchidopexy

Occupational: Exposure to toxic substances including chemicals, radiation

Time away from home through work

Sexual:

Onset of puberty — Libido

Coital habits — Impotence

Premature ejaculation — Use and knowledge of the fertile period

FEMALE

Infertility: Duration of infertility

Length and type of previous contraceptive use

Fertility in previous relationships as well as present liaison

Fertility subsequently, if known, of any former partners

Previous investigations and treatment for infertility

Menstrual: Cyclicity

Pain

Bouts of amenorrhoea

Menorrhagia

Intermenstrual bleeding

Medical: Number of previous pregnancies, including abortions and ectopic pregnancies

Any associated sepsis

Time to initiate previous pregnancies

Surgical: Especially abdominal or pelvic surgery

Sexual: Coital frequency/timing, including knowledge of the fertile period

Investigation of infertility
Examination

MALE

General: Height, weight, body mass index (BMI) and blood pressure

Evidence of hypoandrogenism and gynaecomastia

Groin: Exclude inguinal hernia (patient in upright position)

Palpate testes and note testicular volume, using an orchidometer

Genitalia: Note site in scrotum of testicles

Palpate epididymes for modularity or tenderness

Check presence and normality of vasa deferentia

Check for presence of a possible varicocoele

Examine penis for any structural abnormality, e.g. hypospadias

FEMALE

General: Height, weight, BMI

Fat and hair distribution

Note presence, or absence, of acne and galactorrhoea

Pelvis: Assess state of the hymen

Assess normality of clitoris and labia

Assess vagina, looking for such problems as infection or vaginal septa

Check for presence of cervical polyps

Assess accessibility of the cervix for insemination

Record uterine size, position, mobility and tenderness

Perform cervical smear (if appropriate)

Appropriate initial investigations

MALE

Semen analysis remains the most important facet of male investigation. A minimum of two specimens should be assessed, at least one month apart. It is desirable, in order to avoid unhelpful and frustrating duplication, for GP-referred assessments to take place in the same laboratory which serves the clinic to which the couple may ultimately be referred. It is imperative that clear instructions regarding the method of production and transport of specimens, as well as appropriate advice on the period of abstinence, are given by the laboratory. The production of two specimens minimises the chance of laboratory error, and the likelihood that a transient illness such as influenza might provide a misleading indication of abnormal spermatogenesis. What constitutes a normal result is perhaps a matter for debate. Large laboratories may have their own local population-based normal ranges but, in the absence of such information, the World Health Organization values for definition of normality can be applied (Table 2.1). Additional investigations may be required if the semen analysis fails to meet these criteria.

FEMALE

At the outset it is advisable to ensure that the woman is rubella immune and that she is taking folic acid (0.4 mg/day) to prevent neural tube defects.

The preliminary investigation centres on the need to demonstrate that the woman is ovulating. This is almost certainly the case if she has a regular monthly cycle. Laboratory evidence may be obtained through measurement of serum progesterone in the putative luteal phase of the menstrual cycle. Levels should be in excess of 30 nmol/l seven days after ovulation. For this reason sampling should be arranged for day 21 in the context of a 28-day cycle, with serial checks made beyond this point if the cycle is more prolonged or variable in length. Results should be interpreted only in relation to the onset of the subsequent period. If the level is below 30 nmol/l the test should be repeated in a subsequent cycle. In the absence of any clues in history or examination to suggest the possibility of an endocrine disorder these tests would be sufficient. If, however, there is a history of irregular menstruation, or periods of amenorrhoea, in particular if associated with galactorrhoea, hirsutism or obesity, then additional biochemical tests are appropriate (see Figures 2.1 and 4.1) . There is no evidence that the use of temperature charts and LH detection methods to time intercourse improves outcome and their use should be discouraged.

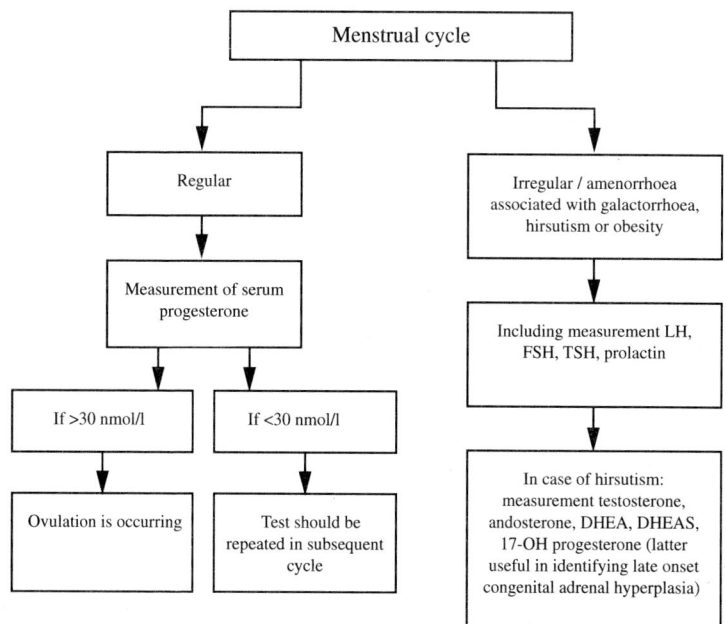

Figure 2.1 Female investigations required in the management of infertility; DHEA = dehydroepiandrosterone, DHEAS = dehydroepiandrosterone sulphate

The investigations outlined above can be initiated by the GP but they also provide the basis for hospital investigation. It is a useful clinical procedure to send the couple a questionnaire to supplement the information provided in the GP's referral letter. Valuable time can then be saved if routine questions in respect of history and previous investigations can be avoided.

KEYPOINTS
- Semen analysis remains the most important male investigation.
- The preliminary investigation centres on a desire to demonstrate that the woman is ovulating.
- If there is a history of irregular menstruation, or periods of amenorrhoea, additional biochemical tests are appropriate.

General advice for practitioners to give to patients

Table 2.2 gives a summary of general advice. There is reasonable evidence to support the suggestion that smoking reduces female fertility, while in men it is known that smoking may affect sperm quality. In men there is

Table 2.2 Summary of general advice given to patients

Advice	Action
Smoking	Advise both partners to stop
Alcohol	Both partners to limit alcohol intake if attempting to conceive
BMI	Encourage women with a body mass index in excess of 30 to lose weight
Temperature	Advise men to wear loose fitting underwear and trousers and avoid conditions that might elevate scrotal temperature

evidence that high alcohol intake can influence reproductive function adversely, as well as general health. There is less convincing evidence linking alcohol and female fertility, but intake in excess of two units per day of alcohol is thought to be detrimental to the fetus in pregnancy. Women with a body mass index in excess of 30 should be encouraged to lose weight, as this may cause a resumption in ovulation, or alternatively enhance the response to treatment where instituted. Hyperthermia is likely to adversely affect sperm quality (see also Chapter 3).

Further tests

FEMALE

Where preliminary investigations suggest that the woman is ovulating and sperm production is satisfactory, pelvic assessment should be undertaken (Table 2.3). Laparoscopy and dye hydrotubation is the investigation of choice, in order to identify those cases with endometriosis and peritubal adhesions. The hysterosalpingogram (HSG) can be helpful in those cases where pelvic pathology has been found at laparoscopy and further information is required to clarify the extent of tubal disease and perhaps the suitability of such patients for tubal surgery.

It is debatable whether assessment of tubal status is necessary in other clinical situations, particularly in women with long-standing, otherwise unexplained, infertility. Present evidence would suggest that minor abnormalities of the uterine cavity such as tubocornual polyps are of little importance in the genesis of infertility. The use of ultrasound in combination with sonoreflective contrast media to visualise intrauterine and tubal pathology has recently been promoted as an alternative outpatient investigation, but has yet to gain widespread popularity. Prospective studies are also awaited to determine whether hysteroscopy may have a part to play in the routine investigation of infertile women,

Table 2.3 Summary of pelvic investigations

Procedure	Comments
Laparoscopy + dye hydrotubation	Investigation of choice Identifies endometriosis and peritubal adhesions
Hysterosalpingogram	Helpful in cases where pelvic pathology found
Ultrasound + sonoreflective contrast media	Used to visualise intrauterine and tubal pathology Yet to gain widespread popularity
Hysteroscopy	Prospective studies awaited May be feasible in women with identified intrauterine abnormalities
Screening for chlamydia	Recommended for women considered at risk Antibiotic prophylaxis may be an alternative Collaboration with a genitourinary clinic advisable

though in women with identified intrauterine abnormalities hysteroscopic surgery may be feasible. Women considered at risk, generally those less than 30 years, should be screened for *Chlamydia trachomatis* before any uterine instrumentation, using an appropriately sensitive technique. Alternatively, antibiotic prophylaxis, for example with doxycycline, may be considered. It is recommended that where chlamydial infection is discovered there should be a local mechanism whereby the disease can be notified and sexual partners treated. Collaboration with a genitourinary clinic is advisable.

MALE

The capacity of sperm to fertilise an egg depends on a complex series of biological events including transport to the site of fertilisation, sperm-egg recognition, the acrosome reaction and fusion of the sperm to the oocyte. It has been claimed that the postcoital test (PCT) is useful in providing information about sperm function in the male (Oei *et al.* 1995). However, systematic review of the literature would suggest that the test lacks validity for routine use. Nevertheless, if sexual dysfunction is suspected, or the male partner cannot or will not provide a semen sample for analysis, the PCT may have a place, even at an early stage in investigations. It is crucial that the test is done at the correct stage in the cycle, i.e. at the time of maximal cervical mucus production prior to ovulation. Inappropriate timing of the test may provide misleading information and cause unnecessary concern. Ideally, mucus production should be assessed daily using an objective method. Occasionally, mucus production may be poor until the day of the beginning of the LH surge and this may indicate a functional problem within the cervix, an unusual situation even in cases where there has been previous cervical surgery. This need for precise timing leads to a sex-on-demand approach to investigation, which may produce additional strain and tension for an already overburdened couple, trying to cope with the stress of their infertility and their associated loss of self-esteem.

Other tests of sperm function, including computerised analysis of sperm-movement characteristics and sperm cervical mucus penetration tests, among others, are not recommended for routine use, nor is the testing for antisperm antibodies in semen. The place for such tests will be discussed in Chapter Three.

KEYPOINTS
- Where preliminary investigations have suggested that the woman is ovulating and sperm production is satisfactory, pelvic assessment should be undertaken.
- Laparoscopy and dye hydrotubation is the investigation of choice.
- If sexual dysfunction is suspected, or the male partner cannot or will not provide a semen sample for analysis, the PCT may have a place at an early stage in investigations.

Conclusion

The preliminary assessment of egg and sperm availability, together with a determination that the gametes can meet, should provide a diagnosis for the majority of couples. In most cases, a prognosis, usually favourable, can be given to the couple. Appropriate therapeutic strategies can be instituted where required, with specialist involvement if necessary. The lines of communication within a regional framework should be set out clearly, with the involvement of GPs intimately linked to the process of assessment. Clinical protocols should be clearly set out in order that unnecessary repetition of investigations is minimised. Clinics should be structured so that the same practitioner sees patients as far as possible and if subspecialist help is required this should be readily available. Information leaflets are a valuable adjunct to the smooth running of the clinic and suitably trained nursing staff should be an integral part of the service, providing a day-to-day focus for patient contact. Such personnel can plan and co-ordinate treatment protocols on an individual basis and, linked to a sympathetic counselling service, will be able to best serve the considerable and complex needs of the infertile population entrusted to their care.

References and recommended reading

Hamilton, M.P.R. (1992) The initial assessment of the infertile couple. *Current Obstetrics and Gynaecology* **2**, 2–7

Oei, S.G., Helmerhorst, F.M. and Keirse, M.J. (1995) When is the postcoital test normal? A critical appraisal. *Hum Reprod* **10**, 1711–14

Royal College of Obstetricians and Gynaecologists (1998a) *The Initial Investigation and Management of the Infertile Couple.* London: RCOG Press (Evidence-based Clinical Guidelines No. 2)

Royal College of Obstetricians and Gynaecologists (1998b) *The Management of Infertility in Secondary Care.* London: RCOG Press (Evidence-based Clinical Guidelines No. 3)

Vessey, M.P., Wright, N.M., McPherson, K. *et al.* (1978) Fertility after stopping different forms of contraception. *BMJ* **i**, 265–7

3 Male factor infertility

Introduction

Male factor infertility is responsible for up to 25% of all cases of infertility and may contribute in a further 25%. Few advances have been made in understanding the aetiology or prevention of male factor infertility. However, with the advent of assisted reproduction techniques, in particular the use of intracytoplasmic sperm injection (ICSI), men with severe oligozoospermia and many with azoospermia have a chance to father their own children. ICSI provides symptomatic treatment and does not cure the condition. For the present, ICSI is the best option, although it does not address the underlying condition (see Chapter 8).

Aetiology

Most men presenting with infertility cannot be given an explanation as to the cause of the problem nor can a demonstrable pathology be identified. A study published by the World Health Organization (1992) found no demonstrable cause in almost 50% of couples with male-factor infertility. The distribution of diagnoses when male-factor subfertility was encountered in the WHO study are shown in Table 3.1.

VARICOCOELE

A varicocoele is a state of varicosity of the testicular veins. The veins of the pampiniform plexus are dilated and tortuous producing a swelling that feels like a 'bag of worms' (Figure 3.1). The clinical significance of varicocoele in the context of male infertility remains controversial since it is a common clinical finding among both normal and infertile men, occurring in 5–20% of the general population and 10–40% of the infertile population. Most varicocoeles are asymptomatic but some may cause a dragging pain on the affected side. Varicocoeles are usually found coincidentally during investigation of the male partner of a couple presenting with subfertility (Table 3.2) and are classified as primary (idiopathic) or secondary.

Table 3.1　Causes of male factor infertility[a]

Cause	Incidence (%)
No demonstrable cause	48.8
Varicocoele	12.6
Idiopathic oligozoospermia	11.2
Accessory gland infection	6.9
Idiopathic teratozoospermia	5.9
Idiopathic asthenozoospermia	3.9
Isolated seminal plasma abnormalities	3.5
Suspected immunological subfertility	3.0
Congenital abnormalities	1.7
Systemic diseases	1.4
Sexual inadequacy	1.3
Obstructive azoospermia	0.9
Idiopathic necrozoospermia	0.8
Ejaculatory inadequacy	0.7
Hyperprolactinaemia	0.6
Iatrogenic causes	0.5
Karyotype abnormalities	0.1
Partial obstruction to ejaculatory duct	0.1
Retrograde ejaculation	0.1
Immotile cilia syndrome	< 1.0
Pituitary lesions	< 1.0
Gonadotrophin deficiency	< 1.0

[a]Source: World Health Organization survey (Rowe *et al*. 1993)

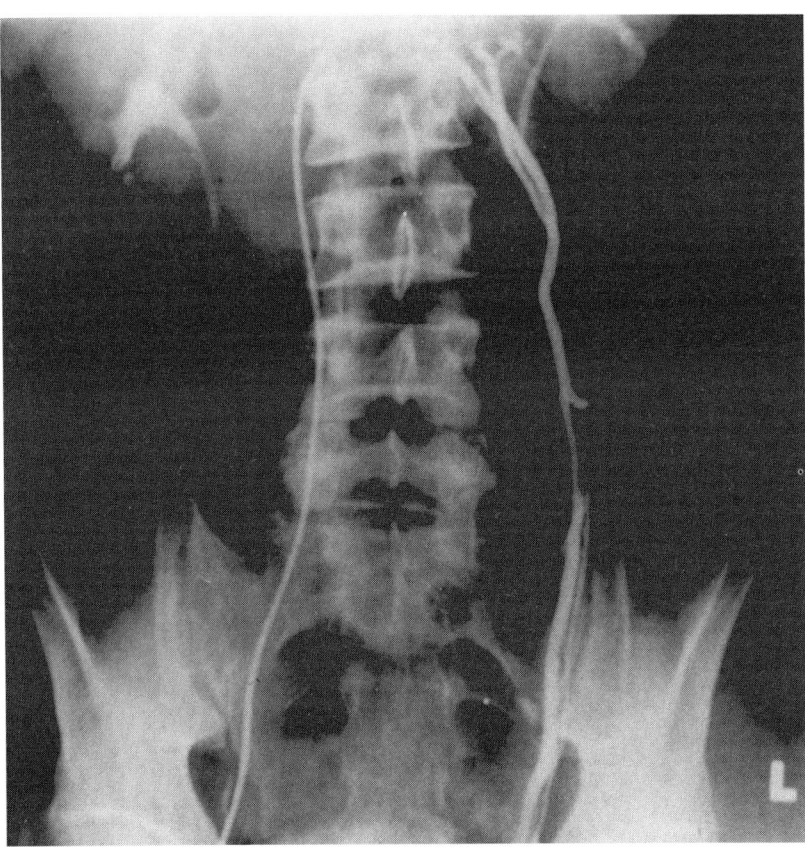

Figure 3.1   X-ray of embolism of left-sided varicocoele

Table 3.2   Categorisation of varicocoeles on physical examination

Category	Description
Subclinical	No varicocoele at clinical examination but present on scrotal thermography or Doppler ultrasonography
Grade 1	No visible or palpable distension except on valsalva manoeuvre
Grade 2	Intrascrotal venous distension only palpable not visible
Grade 3	Distended venous plexus bulges through scrotal skin and easily palpable

- Primary or idiopathic varicocoeles are most common and thought to be due to:
  - compression of the left renal vein between the aorta and the superior mesenteric artery (the nutcracker phenomenon)
  - insufficiency of the valves in the left testicular vein causing reflux of blood from the venocaval circulation down the left testicular vein to the pampiniform plexus of the testis and, through anastomosis, with the cremasteric plexus into the external iliac veins.
- Secondary varicocoeles are rare and may occur due to obstruction of the left testicular vein by a growth like a hypernephroma along the renal veins. Characteristically, these varicocoeles do not decompress in the supine position.

Most varicocoeles are left-sided and associated with reduced testicular volume. Testicular volume correlates with sperm concentration in both fertile and infertile men (World Health Organization 1992). WHO suggests that there is an inverse relationship between semen quality and the presence and severity of varicocoeles, at least among the male partners of infertile couples, and varicocoeles are associated with impaired testicular function and infertility. Surgical treatment can involve ligation of the spermatic vein or embolisation.

It has been suggested that surgical treatment of clinically detectable varicocoele in men with oligozoospermia will improve sperm quality and pregnancy rates, but there is little evidence to support this. It is also unclear whether treatment of a varicocoele in men with normal sperm counts will increase fertility rates.

HYPOGONADOTROPHIC HYPOGONADISM

This rare condition may be caused by either hypothalamic or pituitary failure and can be congenital or acquired. Patients usually present with clinical evidence of androgen deficiency with the condition often being recognised around the time of puberty. However, adult onset (post-pubertal) hypogonadotrophic hypogonadism may be recognised in males presenting with infertility due to trauma, tumour, chronic inflammatory lesions or iron overload.

In the congenital type a complete absence of gonadotrophin-releasing hormone (GnRH) results in the absence of secondary sexual development and total testicular failure, males having small, atrophic testes. However, males with a less severe or partial deficiency will have less profound manifestations of the disorder, with larger but yet underdeveloped testes. Most of these patients will have anosmia or hyposmia (Kallman syndrome).

Low or undetectable levels of gonadotrophins (LH and FSH) which lead to lack of spermatogenesis and low testosterone levels usually confirm the diagnosis.

COITAL DYSFUNCTION

Causes of coital dysfunction are shown in Table 3.3. Psychosexual dysfunction as a primary cause of male infertility is uncommon, although it can occur after prolonged investigations and treatment of infertility and may lead to sexual or ejaculatory dysfunction.

The incidence of hyperprolactinaemia in impotent men ranges from 1–5%. Endocrine disorders such as androgen deficiency and hypothy-

Table 3.3   Aetiology of coital dysfunction

Problem	Results from
Ejaculatory failure	Spinal cord injury
	Medical disorders:
	– multiple sclerosis
	– diabetes mellitus
	– chronic renal failure
	Bladder-neck surgery
	Retroperitoneal lymph node dissection
Erectile or ejaculatory problems	Depression
	Alcohol abuse
	Medication:
	– adrenergic blocking agents
	– antihypertensive agents
	– psychotrophic agents
	Psychosexual
Loss of libido and impotence	Hyperprolactinaemia due to:
	– pituitary adenomas
	– chronic renal failure
	– idiopathic
	– drug therapy
Retrograde ejaculation	Transurethral prostatectomy
	Retroperitoneal lymph-node dissection
	Diabetic neuropathy due to:
	– injury to the lumbar sympathetic nerves
	– damage to the neck of the bladder

roidism can also lead to coital dysfunction but usually present with the clinical manifestations of the specific disorder.

In patients with pituitary adenoma, symptoms such as impotence and loss of libido often precede other manifestations of the disorder. Imaging of the hypothalamo-pituitary axis is mandatory in all patients with sexual dysfunction and elevated prolactin levels.

Retrograde ejaculation is the propulsion of seminal fluid from the posterior urethra into the bladder. A diagnosis can be made by the absence of ejaculate (aspermia) and by the presence of a large number of spermatozoa in post-masturbatory urine.

IMMUNOLOGICAL CAUSES

Antisperm antibodies may be present in serum, in the seminal plasma or bound to spermatozoa and have been associated with infertility, although the significance of their role remains unclear. Antisperm antibodies are usually immunoglobulins of the IgG or IgA isotypes and can be bound to various sites on the spermatozoa (head, midpiece, tail or combinations thereof). Significant risk factors for the development of antisperm antibodies include vasectomy reversal and prior infection such as epididymitis, sexually transmitted diseases and orchitis. About 70% of males have antisperm antibodies after vasectomy and this is of clinical importance if reversal is required.

The presence of antisperm antibodies may have a detrimental effect on fertility by affecting sperm motility causing:

- destruction of gametes
- acrosomal reaction abnormalities
- inhibition of zona pellucida binding
- prevention of embryo cleavage and early development of the embryo.

GENITAL TRACT INFECTION

Acute clinical infections of the genital tract (orchitis, epididymis, prostatovesiculitis or urethritis) may present with fever, pain, decreased sexual activity and may cause decreased semen quality or temporary obstruction of the genital tract. Gram negative enterococci, chlamydia and gonococcus have all been associated with clinical infection. Transmission of acute infections to the female partner may lead to pelvic inflammatory disease and its sequelae, which includes tubal occlusion and infertility. Acute bacterial infections of the genital tract or venereal diseases can lead to infection of the accessory glands resulting in permanent structural damage and scarring, with obstruction to the outflow tract. Where such infection exists it should be treated with antibiotics. There is no evidence to suggest that antibiotic use will improve impaired male infertility.

Symptomatic orchitis occurs in 27–30% of males over 11 years of age who are diagnosed with mumps. In 17% of cases it is bilateral. The prevalence of infertility after viral orchitis is unknown but impaired fertility occurs in bilateral orchitis due to seminiferous tubular atrophy and impairment of spermatogenesis.

GENITAL TRACT OBSTRUCTION

The most common cause of genital tract obstruction is iatrogenic following vasectomy. Other causes of obstruction to the outflow tract, such as postinfective blocks, should be suspected in patients with azoospermia or oligozoospermia with normal-size testis. Success rates after surgery depends on the skill of the surgeon and the site of obstruction; epididymovasostomy for a block in the caudal part of the epididymis has better success than one in the capital part.

Ejaculatory duct obstruction is a rare cause of obstructive azoospermia and is commonly caused by congenital malformations.

TESTICULAR MALDESCENT

Failure of the hypothalamic-pituitary gonadal axis may be associated with failure of testicular descent. Maldescended testis occurs in 3–6% of males at birth.

The abnormal position of the testis should be corrected by the end of the first year as germ-cell degeneration and dysplasia begins early in life, resulting in irreversible testicular damage and infertility. There is also a five- to ten-fold increase in the risk of malignancy in the undescended testis. In addition to improving spermatogenesis, orchidopexy prevents malignant change, trauma and torsion and improves psychological effects.

CHROMOSOMAL ABNORMALITIES

The most common chromosomal disorder that interferes with spermatogenesis is Klinefelter syndrome (47XXY). Fifteen percent of azoospermic men and 4% of oligozoospermic men have an abnormal chromosomal karyotype. An incidence of 2.2% of chromosomal abnormalities was detected in over 2000 men attending a male subfertility clinic over a ten-year period.

Other chromosomal abnormalities that may be found in the infertile male population include reciprocal X or Y autosomal translocations, as well as XYY and XX males. Males with azoospermia or severe oligo-zoospermia should have a karyotype.

CHEMOTHERAPY, RADIOTHERAPY AND TOXINS

Treatment with certain drugs or exposure to radiation or chemicals can affect actively dividing germ cells causing defective spermatogenesis, which may be temporary or permanent.

Table 3.4 shows a list of drugs that interfere with spermatogenesis. Anabolic steroids used by some athletes can interfere with feedback to the pituitary, causing a reduction in gonadotrophin secretion. This results in testicular atrophy, which is reversible.

Cytotoxic drugs used for the treatment of testicular cancer, Hodgkin's disease, non-Hodgkin's lymphoma and leukaemia may have a deleterious affect on fertility. The disease itself can also cause infertility. Cytotoxic treatment damages differentiating spermatogonia with most patients becoming azoospermic within eight weeks of commencing treatment. Alkylating agents may cause irreversible damage.

Exposure to radiation destroys germ cells with irreversible arrests of spermatogenesis, which invariably results in sterility.

Additionally, toxins in the workplace and environment may cause damage to the germ cells. A well-documented example is the chemical

Table 3.4	Therapeutic drugs interfering with male fertility (Rowe et al. 1993)
Drug	*Action*
Cancer chemotherapy	Alkylating agents cause irreversible damage.
Hormone treatment	High-dose corticosteroids, androgens, anti-androgens, oestrogens and LHRH agonist
Cimetidine	May competitively inhibit androgen effect on the receptor
Sulphasalazine	Can cause impairment of sperm quality by direct toxicity
Spironolactone	Antagonises the action of androgen in some tissue
Nitrofurantoin	May cause impairment of sperm quality by direct toxicity
Niradozole	May cause temporary depression of spermatogenesis in man
Colchicine	Causes depression of fertility by direct toxicity to spermatogenesis

dibromochloropropane (BMCP) which caused azoospermia in 14 of 25 non-vasectomised men in a Californian pesticide factory.

IDIOPATHIC MALE INFERTILITY

Up to 50% of those with male factor subfertility have no demonstrable cause. A diagnosis of idiopathic infertility can only be made after all other causes of infertility have been excluded. Semen analysis may show varying degrees of abnormality and may be associated with elevated serum FSH, indicating failure of spermatogenesis.

KEYPOINTS

- Varicocoeles are associated with impaired testicular function and infertility.
- Psychosexual dysfunction as a primary cause of male infertility is uncommon.
- Imaging of the hypothalamo-pituitary axis is mandatory in all patients with sexual dysfunction and elevated prolactin levels.
- About 70% of males have antisperm antibodies after vasectomy and this is of clinical importance if reversal is required.
- The most common cause of genital-tract obstruction is iatrogenic following vasectomy.
- Maldescended testis occurs in 3–6% of males at birth and should be corrected by the end of the first year.
- Males with azoospermia or severe oligozoospermia should have a karyotype.
- Up to 50% of those with male factor subfertility have no demonstrable cause.

CLINICAL MANAGEMENT

Both partners should be involved in the management. It is important to take other factors like female age, duration of infertility and previous pregnancy into consideration when managing a couple with suboptimal spermatogenesis.

HISTORY AND EXAMINATION

A detailed history should be obtained from the male. It is important to enquire about previous infertility investigations undertaken in order to avoid repetition and save time and resources.

The male partner should be examined clinically, as described in Chapter 2.

Investigations

SEMEN ANALYSIS

Two semen analyses should have been performed during initial investigations (see Chapter 2). These can be arranged in primary care. The RCOG (1998a) evidence-based clinical guideline on the initial investigation of the infertile couple recommends that: 'Laboratories that perform semen analysis should undertake this according to recognised WHO methodology. Laboratories should also perform internal quality control and belong to an external quality control scheme'.

If the semen analysis is abnormal or there is cause for concern in the history or clinical examination, further investigations of the male partner should be undertaken in a secondary or tertiary centre (see Table 2.1 for normal levels).

ENDOCRINE TESTS

Endocrine tests (Figure 3.2) include:

- serum FSH
- serum testosterone
- prolactin.

Serum FSH

Serum FSH should be measured in the male partner with azoospermia or severe oligozoospermia ($\leqslant 5$ M/ml sperm density). It has virtually replaced testicular biopsy in differentiating between an obstructive azoospermia and non-obstructive or secretory azoospermia (failure of spermatogenesis).

In obstructive azoospermia spermatogenesis is normal. In non-obstructive or secretory azoospermia there is failure of spermatogenesis.

FSH estimation may in addition give prognostic information in men prior to testicular biopsy if ICSI is being considered, although this does not totally exclude the possibility of sperm recovery.

Serum testosterone

Serum testosterone is only indicated if hypogonadism is suspected. Males with hypogonadism of hypothalamic or pituitary origin will have low FSH and low testosterone.

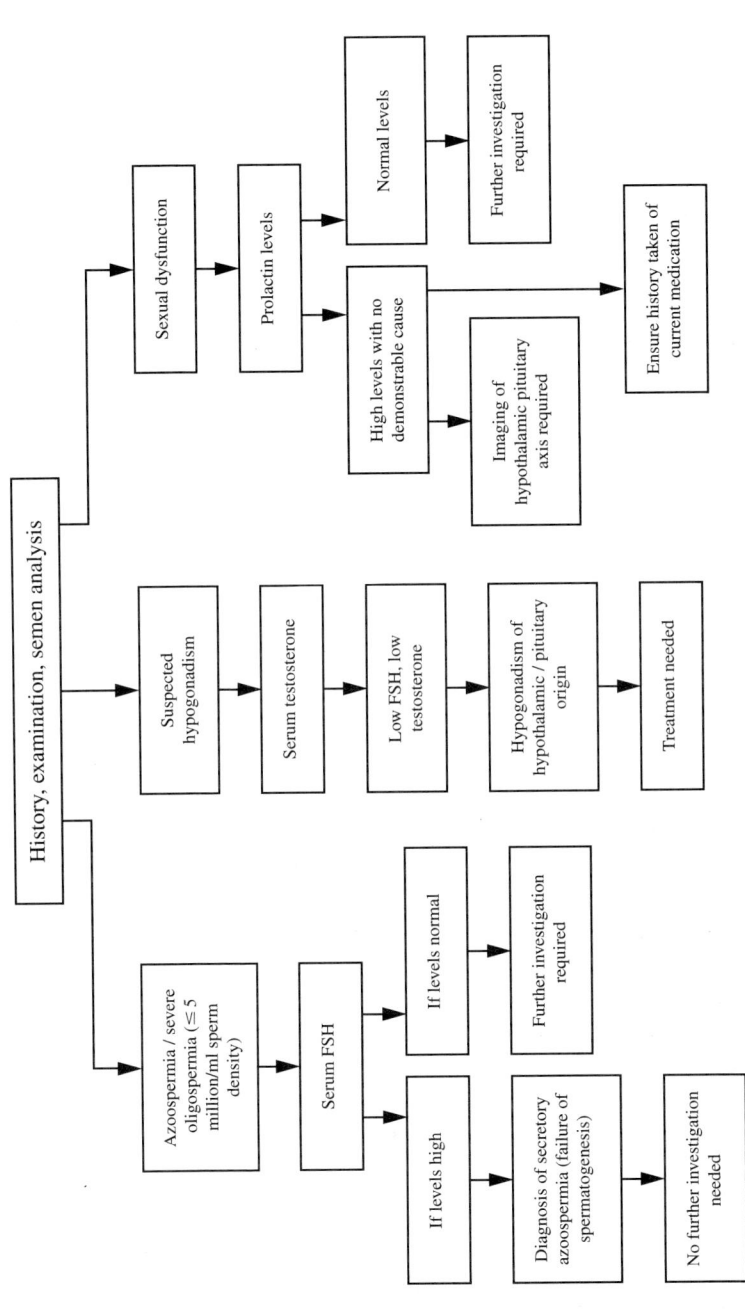

Figure 3.2 Endocrine tests used in the investigation of male infertility

Prolactin

Virtually all men with hyperprolactinaemia have sexual dysfunction and it is mandatory to check for elevated prolactin levels in men complaining of loss of libido and impotence. Imaging of the hypothalamic-pituitary axis is indicated in males with high prolactin levels with no demonstrable cause to detect tumours such as prolactinomas, craniopharyngiomas or tumours compressing the pituitary stalk.

It should be borne in mind that elevated prolactin levels might also occur in men on medications such as tranquillisers and sulpiride (Figure 3.1).

MICROBIOLOGICAL ASSESSMENT OF SEMEN

The biological significance of the presence of white blood cells in semen and asymptomatic subclinical infection is unclear. Many organisms are urethral contaminants of doubtful clinical significance. An increased number of leucocytes in the ejaculate during routine semen analysis are an indication for culture to be performed although this does not always indicate infection. Semen culture should be performed in males with microscopic evidence of infections as well as those with symptoms of orchitis, epididymitis or prostatitis. Male partners of women with acute tubal disease should also be screened. Microbiological assessment may be indicated prior to intrauterine insemination although infective complications following intrauterine insemination are rare.

IMAGING OF THE GENITAL TRACT

Diagnostic tests of varicocoele

Varicocoele can be diagnosed by thermography, ultrasound with Doppler blood flow (higher false positive), radionuclide angiography (higher false negative) or retrograde venography. The latter is the gold standard test, although it is invasive.

Scrotal ultrasound scan

This is not performed routinely but should be undertaken if testicular tumours are suspected. In addition, an ultrasound may be helpful in detecting hydrocoeles and epididymal cysts etc. and may be better than clinical examination.

Vasography

This is performed in patients with obstruction to the vas deferens and usually takes place in theatre prior to surgery, in order to detect the site of obstruction.

IN VITRO TESTS OF SPERM FUNCTION

The ESHRE Andrology Special Interest Group (1996) reviewed four areas of advanced diagnostic andrology, identified as 'research tests' by WHO. These were:

- computer-assisted sperm analysis (CASA)
- zona-free hamster egg penetration test (HEPT)
- acrosome reaction testing
- zona binding test (ZBT)

The RCOG (1998b) evidence-based clinical guideline on the management of infertility in secondary care recommends that: 'Certain *in vitro* tests of sperm function can be of use in predicting fertility. However, at this stage their use and interpretation should be restricted to those few centres with relevant expertise'. It is likely that two of the above tests, CASA and HEPT, will be upgraded to optional tests in the new edition of the WHO manual.

Computer-assisted sperm analysis

In this technique, a computer processes electrical signals of sperm motility obtained by a video camera attached to a microscope, either by direct analysis of the signals or by analysis from videotape. CASA systems can obtain information on sperm density and motility including the vigour and pattern of individual spermatozoa movements.

WHO recommends the use of the haemocytometer to measure sperm concentration since the computer may be inaccurate due to the presence of cellular elements and particulate matter which look similar to spermatozoa.

Using the CASA system to measure sperm motility may also be inaccurate since the system defines motile sperm as the threshold of forward velocity while visual perception of motility is by the presence of flagellar activity irrespective of forward motility. Hence, WHO recommends that direct visual inspection should be carried out to measure the percentage of motile sperm in addition to the CASA system.

CASA should be able to provide an increase in repeatability and reliability between technicians and to provide quantitative data predictive of *in vivo* and *in vitro* fertility. Data generated by CASA have been shown to be significantly associated with time to conception *in vivo*.

It is unlikely that a single sperm function test like CASA will be able to predict fertility and it is likely to be used in conjunction with other sperm-function tests.

Zona-free hamster egg penetration test

The acrosome reaction occurs due to interaction between the sperm plasma membrane and a glycoprotein constituent of the zona pellucida. Sperm-oocyte fusion does not take place in the absence of an acrosomal reaction.

The conventional HEPT (type I protocols) requires prolonged periods of incubation for the acrosomal reaction and capacitation to occur spontaneously and has high false negative results.

To avoid prolonged incubation and provide a physiological stimulus to induce the acrosomal reaction and to improve the sensitivity of the assay the intracellular signals can be induced artificially with the divalent cation ionophore A23187. Here the acrosomal reaction is induced artificially in more or less capacitated sperm.

Should the HEPT be conducted correctly with adequate standardisation of techniques among laboratories, the test correlates well with IVF results, especially in conjunction with sperm morphology. Additionally, HEPT could be considered an optional test of sperm function in the clinical situation, and those laboratories with a proven record of good assay repeatability may perform it.

Testicular biopsy

Testicular biopsy was initially used as a diagnostic tool to differentiate between obstructive and non-obstructive azoospermia and this has now been replaced by serum FSH measurements.

Testicular biopsy should be carried out only in tertiary centres, which have trained staff and facilities for sperm recovery and cryopreservation (RCOG 1998). Sperm recovered during biopsy can be used for IVF, combined with ICSI, giving the opportunity for azoospermic men to father their own genetic offspring. Cryopreservation facilities should be available since sperm recovered may not be used for ICSI immediately.

Additionally, should sperm extraction not be carried out at the same time as the biopsy this may affect future attempts at sperm recovery due to the possibility of:

- reduction in testicular mass
- trauma causing devascularisation
- fibrosis
- an auto-immune response.

GENETIC STUDIES

Karyotyping

Males with azoospermia or severe oligozoospermia should be karyotyped. Klinefelter syndrome is the most common chromosomal abnormality (46XXY) detected in this group.

Cystic fibrosis screen

The condition of congenital bilateral absence of the vas deferens (CBAVD) is, in the majority of patients, related to defects in the cystic fibrosis transmembrane conductance regulator (CFTR) gene. CBAVD is frequently associated with heterozygosity for the common cystic fibrosis gene (DF 508). A mutation analysis should be performed in males with CBAVD as well as the female partner, since the children have an increased risk of being born with cystic fibrosis and/or CBAVD.

ANTISPERM ANTIBODIES

Tests for antisperm antibodies are not routinely performed. The presence of agglutination, where motile spermatozoa stick to each other, may be suggestive of the presence of antisperm antibodies.

If tests are done they should be performed on a fresh semen sample and can be used for detection and quantification of antibodies. The two screening tests used are:

- mixed agglutinin test (MAR): red blood cells coated with IgA or sensitised with IgG are mixed with non-specific antibody to IgA or IgG (anti-IgA or anti-IgG) and then incubated with the patient's sperm. Sperm with antisperm antibodies will adhere to treated red blood cells
- immunobead test (IBT): this involves using micron-sized polyacrylamide beads with covalently bound antihuman IgA and IgG antibodies. Spermatozoa with beads attached give a positive reaction and the region of binding can also be noted (head, midpiece, tail and mixed).

POSTCOITAL TEST

The postcoital testing of cervical mucus for the presence of progressively motile sperm remains controversial. Since its first introduction in 1866 various infertility treatments have been used in women with abnormal test results. Intrauterine insemination is the recent favourite. However, current evidence suggests that the routine use of the postcoital test leads to more tests and treatments but no significant effect on the pregnancy rate. The postcoital test is a poor predictor of fertility and it is difficult to justify this test as an essential procedure in standard infertility investigations.

Treatment

GENERAL MANAGEMENT

Men who smoke should be advised to stop smoking and those who consume alcohol heavily should be advised to cut down on drinking since these factors can affect reproductive function. Males with a suboptimal semen analysis may be advised to wear loose fitting underwear and avoid conditions that increase the testicular temperature, although more recently the value of this advice has been questioned.

MANAGEMENT OF SPECIFIC CONDITIONS

Varicocoele

In the light of current evidence there is no justification for treating men with a clinically detectable varicocoele with normal sperm counts since this does not improve pregnancy rates. The evidence for treating oligozoospermic men is uncertain and benefit is far from clear.

The surgical procedure that is usually undertaken is to ligate the spermatic vein above the inguinal ligament at the internal inguinal ring. Only occasionally is a local excision indicated in cases where ligation leaves a group of tortuous varicosities. Alternatively, embolisation can be undertaken through a cannula inserted by the femoral or jugular route.

Gonadotrophin deficiency

Hypogonadotrophic hypogonadism is one of the few conditions in the male which can be very successfully treated with restoration of steroidogenesis and spermatogenesis. As with other endocrine-deficiency states, exogenous replacement of the deficient hormone is effective, in this case with the use of gonadotrophin (Table 3.5).

Table 3.5 Summary of gonadotrophin deficiency management

Treatment	Deficiency	Action	Administered as
hCG (source of LH activity)	Acquired hypogonadotrophic hypogonadism (HH)	Stimulates Leydig cells to produce testosterone	Intramuscular injection × 3/week
hCG + hMG (source of FSH)	Acquired/prepubertal HH	As above and causes maturation and proliferation of the germinal cells; stimulates spermatogenesis	Intramuscular injection × 3/week
hCG + highly purified FSH (better tolerated)	Acquired/prepubertal HH	Effective in stimulating spermatogenesis and steroidogenesis	Self-administered subcutaneously over months/years to achieve maximum testicular size and spermatogenesis
Pulsatile GnRH therapy	HH of hypothalamic origin	Stimulation of the pituitary and testis; stimulates spermatogenesis	Battery-driven portable infusion pump; administers set dose subcutaneously (worn continuously approx. l year)
Dopamine agonists (bromocriptine)	HH due to prolactinomas (causing hyperprolactinaemia)	Normalises serum prolactin levels, LH secretion begins, testosterone levels normalise, restoration of potency and fertility	5–10 mg/day in divided doses

Treatment with exogenous gonadotrophins or GnRH therapy can result in effective spermatogenesis in 70–90% of men who become fertile, even with sperm counts well below normal limits. Once fertility has been achieved treatment can be substituted with testosterone in the form of oral, injectables or implants.

Ejaculatory problems

Counselling forms an important part in the management of couples with psychosexual dysfunction. Various methods of semen procurement such as external vibratory massage, intrathecal injection of neostigmine, direct aspiration of sperm from the vas and electroejaculation have been tried in patients with erectile and ejaculatory dysfunction. Rectal probe electroejaculation has become an accepted method to procure sperm with successful sperm recovery in > 80% in experienced centres. Sperm procured from electroejaculation can be used for intrauterine insemination (IUI) or IVF.

The sperm quality following electroejaculation is usually poor, with a high sperm count and usually normal morphology but low motility. The possible aetiologies for low sperm motility include:

- stasis of seminal fluid
- testicular hyperthermia
- recurrent urinary tract infections
- antisperm antibodies
- urinary contamination due to retrograde ejaculation
- (possibly) effects of heat and electric current generated by electro-ejaculation.

This can probably be overcome with IVF and IVF/ICSI. At present it is not possible to estimate pregnancy rates with a combination of electro-ejaculation and assisted reproductive technology in view of the small number of patients.

The efficacy of medical treatment of retrograde ejaculation is disputable since no randomised controlled trials have been conducted to determine efficacy. Medical treatment for reversal of retrograde ejaculation facilitates antegrade ejaculation by stimulating peristalsis in the vas deferens and closing the bladder neck. This may be achieved by either increasing sympathetic tone at the bladder neck or by decreasing parasympathetic activity. Drugs used are shown in Table 3.6.

Viagra® (sildenafil) (Pfizer) has recently gained a high profile. Until recently available therapy for erectile dysfunction included:

- implants
- intracavernosal injection

Table 3.6 Drugs included in treatment of retrograde ejaculation

Alpha-adrenergic agonists
   Phenylpropanolamine hydrochloride 25 mg orally twice daily
   Oxedrine 15–60 mg in a single intravenous dose

Anticholinergics
   Brompheniramine maleate 8 mg twice daily
   Imipramine in a daily dose of 25–50 mg

- intraurethral pellets
- vacuum devices
- sex therapy.

The pathway for sexual arousal and stimulation leading to erection is the production of cyclic guanosine monophosphate (GMP) in the corpus cavernosum, which relaxes the smooth muscle and causes blood to fill the corpora. Sildenafil specifically inhibits the isoenzyme cyclic GMP specific phosphodiesterase type five, which is responsible for the breakdown of cyclic GMP in the corpus cavernosum. Hence, it produces sexual arousal or stimulation similar to a 'natural' erectile response. Although orgasmic function, satisfaction with intercourse and overall sexual function is improved, it has no effect on sexual drive.

Sildenafil is administered in a dose of 30–60 mg. Common adverse effects include headache, flushing, dyspepsia, nasal congestion and transient disturbance of colour discrimination. Other serious adverse effects include priapism and it can potentiate the hypotensive effect of nitrates.

Immunological infertility

The majority of trials evaluating the role of steroids in the treatment of antisperm antibodies are uncontrolled and the randomised controlled trials are methodologically flawed. Adverse effects of steroids include dyspepsia, facial flushing, bloating, irritability, skin rashes and Cushingoid appearance with rare serious complications such as bilateral aseptic necrosis of the hip and the risk of severe chickenpox in an unexposed individual.

Due to the potentially serious adverse effects of steroids and conflicting evidence of benefit their use can only be recommended in the context of further research. Patients with high levels of IgA or IgG antibodies should be directly referred for ICSI.

Genital tract obstruction

Reported success rates for vasectomy reversal vary from 17–82%. Factors which influence success rates include:

- type of vasectomy performed
- type of reversal
- surgical technique (macro- or microsurgery)
- presence of other pathology such as varicocoeles or antisperm antibodies
- the experience and skill of the surgeon
- time since vasectomy.

The last two factors are the most important, surgical skill being important for microsurgical techniques.

The longer the time interval from vasectomy to reversal the lower the chance of a successful pregnancy due to the risk of secondary epididymal obstruction.

A cost effectiveness analysis in the USA showed that the most cost-effective approach to the treatment of postvasectomy infertility is microsurgical reversal. This treatment also has the highest chance of resulting in delivery of a child for a single intervention with a delivery rate of 47%, whereas after one cycle of sperm retrieval and ICSI the delivery rate is around 30%. Vasectomy reversal has, in addition, added advantages over ICSI, including the possibility of further pregnancies without further intervention, conception following normal intercourse and avoidance of ovarian hyperstimulation and multiple pregnancy.

Reversal of vasectomy should be the first line of treatment in patients wishing fertility after vasectomy and at present microsurgical epididymal sperm aspiration and ICSI should be reserved for failed surgery or in patients where surgical reconstruction is not feasible.

Obstructive lesions of the genital tract are not a common cause of infertility and reconstructive surgical treatment should only be undertaken by trained surgeons with microsurgical skills in specialist centres with facilities for microsurgery, sperm retrieval and cryostorage.

EMPIRICAL TREATMENT, INCLUDING TREATMENT NOT YET SHOWN TO BE EFFECTIVE

Gonadotrophins

hCG/hMG has been used successfully in males with hypogonadotrophic hypogonadism and this led to its use in idiopathic male infertility. However, there is no evidence to recommend gonadotrophin treatment for idiopathic male infertility.

Gonadotrophin-releasing hormone

GnRH has been used in males with subnormal semen parameters but did not improve semen parameters in idiopathic male infertility.

Androgens

Testosterone is required for normal spermatogenesis and this led to the use of androgens (e.g. mesterolone) in the treatment of idiopathic male infertility, but there is no evidence to support the effectiveness of this treatment. Furthermore, oral doses of testosterone required to achieve serum levels equivalent to intratesticular levels can cause hepatotoxicity and will additionally exert a negative feedback effect on the pituitary-gonadal axis, suppressing FSH and LH secretion and thereby adversely affecting spermatogenesis.

Bromocriptine

Bromocriptine has been clearly shown to be beneficial in patients with hyperprolactinaemia with or without hypogonadotrophic hypogonadism, but it does not reduce prolactin levels in normogonadotrophic males and does not improve semen parameters or fertility.

Anti-oestrogens

Clomiphene or tamoxifen have been used commonly for idiopathic male infertility. Many observational studies have shown apparent improvements in sperm concentration and/or motility as well as pregnancy rates. However, review of randomised studies does not provide proof of effectiveness of anti-oestrogens, although a small beneficial effect remains plausible. With the evidence available so far it is difficult to recommend the use of anti-oestrogens for the treatment of idiopathic male infertility.

Kallikrein

Kallikrein is a glycoprotein, which causes release of kinins from kininogens. Although the mechanism of action of kallikrein is unclear it has been suggested that a local increase in kinins at the testicular level influences spermatogenesis. *In vitro* studies have shown that kallikrein aids sperm motility and improves cervical mucus penetration. Following these observations kallikrein was used in the treatment of idiopathic male infertility. However, recent randomised controlled studies have not shown any demonstrable benefits and the drug should not be used.

Antioxidants

Antioxidants such as glutathione, vitamin E and vitamin C may improve semen parameters. However, at this stage no recommendations can be given for the use of antioxidants for the treatment of male infertility and this mode of treatment requires further evaluation.

Mast-cell blockers

A small single-blind placebo controlled randomised trial has shown that a mast-cell blocker (tranilast) used in the treatment of severe oligozoospermia had statistically significantly higher pregnancy rates in the treatment group as opposed to the control group. This treatment requires further evaluation.

Alpha blockers

Bunazosin has also been shown to statistically improve sperm concentration and motility although there was no difference in pregnancy rates. Again further studies are needed, as the sample size of this study was too small to detect a significant increase in pregnancy rates with treatment.

ASSISTED REPRODUCTION

Superovulation and intrauterine insemination

Intrauterine insemination with or without ovarian stimulation is an effective treatment even where there are abnormalities of semen parameters, although the pregnancy rates remain low (4–6%). Its use may be justified but results cannot be compared with ICSI.

ICSI

Males with severe sperm abnormalities or non-obstructive azoospermia now have the possibility of fathering their own children. However, it should be kept in mind that ICSI is a symptomatic treatment for male infertility and using ICSI does not cure the condition.

Table 3.7   Prevention of infertility

- Surgical treatment (orchidopexy) is indicated by the end of the first year in males with testicular maldescent should endocrine therapy fail, to prevent irreversible damage

- Infections, particularly chlamydia, should be screened for and treated appropriately to prevent upper tract infection which may lead to pelvic inflammatory disease and its sequelae

- Health advice regarding smoking and alcohol consumption should be given

- Patients should avoid using drugs which cause deterioration of semen parameters and use alternative drugs when available

- Elective cryopreservation of sperm prior to radiotherapy or chemotherapy should be offered

---

Donor insemination

The use of unstimulated cycles should be considered the first line of treatment to avoid multiple pregnancy. The use of gonadotrophin stimulation will increase the pregnancy rate at the expense of increasing the multiple pregnancy rates. Success rate is related to female age and previous history of infertility. An overall pregnancy rate of 10% per cycle for unstimulated cycles should be anticipated.

KEYPOINTS
- The significance of a varicocoele in male infertility is controversial, but treatment is unlikely to be helpful.
- Gonadotrophins for hypogonadotrophic hypogonadism and bromocriptine for hyperprolactinaemia are effective treatments.
- The efficacy of medical treatment of retrograde ejaculation is disputable.
- Systemic steroids cannot be currently recommended for immunological infertility.
- Vasectomy reversal should be considered the first line of treatment in men requesting reversal of sterilisation.
- ICSI is an effective treatment, but exposes the female to the hazards of assisted reproduction and does not cure the underlying male anomaly.

Prevention

Methods of preventing the onset of infertility are shown in Table 3.7.

References

ESHRE Andrology Special Interest Group (1996) Consensus Workshop on Advanced Diagnostic and Andrology Techniques *Hum Reprod* **11**, 1463–79

Rowe, P.J., Comhaire, F.H., Hargreave, T.B. and Mellows, H.J. (1993) *WHO Manual for the Standardised Investigation and Diagnosis of the Infertile Couple.* Cambridge: Cambridge University Press

Royal College of Obstetricians and Gynaecologists (1998a) *The Management of Infertility in Secondary Care.* London: RCOG Press (Evidence-based Clinical Guidelines No. 3)

Royal College of Obstetricians and Gynaecologists (1998b) *The Initial Investigation and Management of the Infertile Couple.* London: RCOG Press (Evidence-based Clinical Guidelines No. 2)

World Health Organization (1992) The influence of varicocoele on parameters of fertility in a large group of men presenting to infertility clinics. *Fertil Steril* **57**, 1289–93

4 Disorders of ovulation

Introduction

Ovulation is crucial to fertility. Anovulation or oligo-ovulation is the principal cause of infertility in about one fifth of all subfertile couples, with other quoted incidences varying from 10% to 50%. There have been considerable advances in the management of ovulation disorders, but there is still in some circumstances a disparity between high rates of successful ovulation induction and pregnancy rates. Some of this may be explained by inadequate investigation of other, including male, factors (Chapter 3). There are also iatrogenic problems with ovulation induction, particularly ovarian hyperstimulation syndrome (OHSS) and multiple gestation. Recently, concern has been raised about an increase in the risk of ovarian malignancy in patients undergoing ovarian stimulation.

Classification of ovulation disorders

Ovulation disorders can be classified on the basis of the anatomical site in the hypothalamic-pituitary-ovarian axis where the deficiency exists.

OVARY

The deficiency may be in the ovary itself (intrinsic ovarian failure). Causes include:
- genetic
    Turner XO
    Turner mosaic XO, XX
    XX gonadal agenesis
- autoimmune
- cytotoxic radiotherapy, chemotherapy
- premature menopause.

HYPOTHALAMUS

The ovary may be secondarily affected by abnormalities of GnRH secretion from the hypothalamus. GnRH is the main regulator of gonadotrophin secretion from the pituitary. This could happen in cases of hyperprolactinaemia and Kallmann syndrome, characterised by a lack of GnRH, anosmia and other congenital abnormalities. Weight loss, excessive exercise and stress may also result in altered GnRH secretion.

PITUITARY

There may be disorders of the pituitary itself, resulting in deficiency of gonadotrophins. These include pituitary tumours or pituitary necrosis and thrombosis. A good example of this is Sheehan's syndrome, which is the result of postpartum pituitary necrosis secondary to the hypovolaemia associated with severe postpartum haemorrhage.

HYPOTHALAMIC-PITUITARY DYSFUNCTION

The oligo-anovulation associated with polycystic ovarian syndrome (PCOS) is due to the hypothalamic-pituitary dysfunction secondary to all the other endocrine disturbances associated with this syndrome.

The WHO classification of ovulatory deficiencies is shown in Table 4.1.

Diagnosis

The choice between the different modes of treatment will depend on the correct identification of the underlying problem. Pointers in the history and clinical examination would determine relevant investigations.

Regular menstruation is strongly suggestive evidence of ovulation, but this is not conclusive. In patients with regular cycles, a day-21 progesterone showing a level of 30 nmol/l or more would confirm ovulation. In patients with irregular cycles (but within 45 days), serial progesterone tracking may be necessary (see Chapter 2). These investigations could be done in a primary care setting.

Early referral to a specialist infertility clinic with access to endocrine laboratory facilities and ultrasonography is advisable in patients over the age of 35 years with oligomenorrhoea and primary or secondary amenorrhoea. Figure 4.1 details the investigations needed in patients with oligomenorrhoea (cycles over 45 days) and primary or secondary amenorrhoea.

When amenorrhoea is due to ovarian failure, as in premature menopause, or due to autoimmune causes, a high FSH level is confirmatory. Other tests to detect autoimmune problems would include a

Table 4.1   The WHO classification of ovulatory deficiencies

Group		Characteristics
I	Hypothalamic pituitary failure (hypothalamic amenorrhoea or hypogonadotrophic hypogonadism)	Low/basal gonadotrophins, normal prolactin and oestrogen deficiency with a failure to bleed after a progestational challenge. Includes amenorrhoea related to stress and weight loss, Kallmann syndrome, isolated gonadotrophin deficiency and idiopathic hypogonadotrophic hypogonadism.
II	Hypothalamic pituitary dysfunction	Normal gonadotrophins and oestrogen levels with anovulatory oligo/amenorrhoea. A classic example of this is polycystic ovarian syndrome
III	Ovarian failure	High levels of gonadotrophins with hypogonadism and low oestrogen levels

complete blood count, tests for rheumatoid factor, antinuclear antibodies, a complete thyroid screen with auto-antibody testing, and tests for adrenal function.

Ovarian biopsy was used in the past to differentiate premature menopause from resistant ovary syndrome, but is obsolete as the histological findings have little influence on the clinical management of the patient and the risks of surgery and peritubal adhesions far outweigh any benefit to the patient.

Drug treatment for ovulation induction

CLOMIPHENE CITRATE

This is the most commonly prescribed drug for ovulation induction and accounts for two-thirds of all the fertility drugs used. It is similar in structure to the synthetic oestrogen, diethylstilboestrol and has been in use since the 1960s.

Mechanism of action

Clomiphene exerts a weak biological oestrogen effect and binds to oestrogen receptors. The hypothalamic-pituitary axis is blinded to the

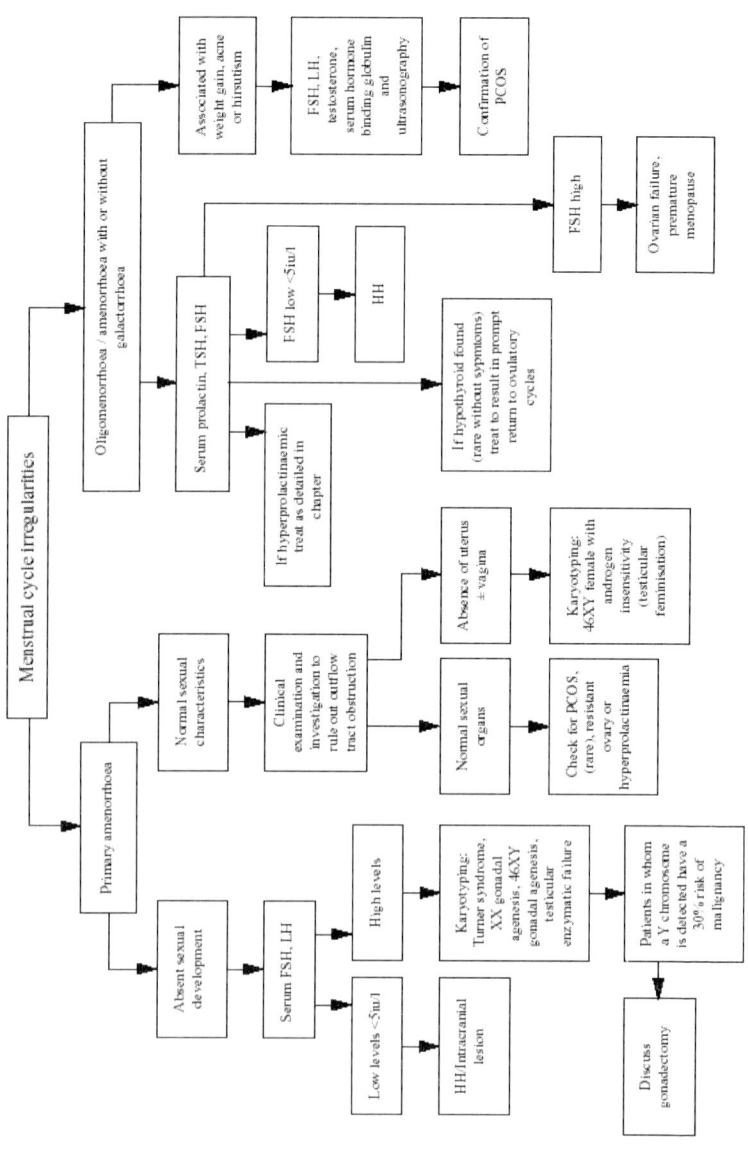

Figure 4.1 Investigations used in the diagnosis of ovulatory disorders

TREATMENT OPTIONS: CONSIDERATIONS

Before embarking on any treatment for ovulation induction, the following should be considered:

- Relevant investigations to make a diagnosis and to select the most appropriate treatment.
- Patient counselling before treatment, especially regarding
    - the risks of ovarian hyperstimulation syndrome
    - multiple pregnancy
    - possibility of fetal reduction
    - putative risk of ovarian cancer.
- Ovulation induction, only if adequate monitoring facilities are available, including free availability of ultrasonography and endocrinology.
- Protocols for reducing the risks, particularly for cancelling cycles to prevent multiple gestations and OHSS.
- Any male factor problems and the results, particularly of a semen analysis.
- Tubal patency, using hysterosalpingography in low-risk women. A laparoscopy and dye transit test is useful if more detailed pelvic examination is desired
    - where endometriosis or pelvic adhesions are suspected
    - if no conception has occurred after six treatment cycles with clomiphene, with ovulation confirmed.
- Advice to women with a BMI over 30 kg/m^2 on the advantages of losing weight prior to therapy. Weight loss not only increases the spontaneous ovulation and pregnancy rates, but also evokes better response to ovulation induction regimens.

DRUGS FOR OVULATION INDUCTION

Anti-oestrogens (clomiphene citrate, tamoxifen)
- used alone
- used in combination with dexamethasone, hMG or hCG

Gonadotrophins (hMG, purified FSH and recombinant FSH)
- used alone
- used in combination with GnRH agonists and antagonists
- low-dose gonadotrophin therapy

GnRH agonists
- used alone (pulsatile administration)
- used in combination with gonadotrophins (as above)

endogenous oestrogen level, which is falsely lowered and negative feed-back is reduced. This signals an increase in GnRH, which in turn leads to an increase in FSH production, which stimulates follicular recruit-ment and growth. Clomiphene also has an anti-oestrogenic action in the uterus, cervix and vagina. Observations suggest that these effects do not appear to be significant in most clinical situations.

An intact hypothalamo-pituitary axis is essential for the effects of clomiphene. It is most useful in:

- normogonadotrophic oligo/amenorrhoeic women
- patients with PCOS with elevated LH to FSH ratios (WHO group II).

Patients with hypogonadotrophic hypogonadism (WHO group 1) and those with ovarian tissue not capable of responding to gonadotrophins (WHO group III) are not suitable for clomiphene.

Treatment regimen

Treatment regimens should be started with the lowest dose which can achieve ovulation. This is generally assumed to be 50 mg orally every day for five days from day two to day six of the menstrual cycle. Occasion-ally, in patients exceptionally sensitive to clomiphene, a 25 mg dose may be adequate. In amenorrhoeic patients, once a pregnancy is ruled out and oestradiol (E_2) and progesterone levels are basal, treatment may be started with or without a progesterone-induced withdrawal bleed.

The patient is assessed for adverse effects and ovulation checked with a luteal phase progesterone estimation. The risk of multiple pregnancy and the variable response of patients to different doses of clomiphene makes it is necessary to monitor at least the first clomiphene cycle with ultrasonography. A luteal phase progesterone estimation alone will not differentiate between uni- and multifollicular ovulation. By using ultra-sound monitoring it is possible to identify those patients who either do not develop a dominant follicle in response to clomiphene, and therefore need an increased dose in the next cycle, from those who produce mul-tiple follicles and need to have their dose reduced. If there is no response to the 50 mg dose, it is increased to 100 mg daily and then possibly to 150 mg. Most centres stop at this dose and move on to other treatment regimens, but doses up to 250 mg have been used. The couple are advised to have intercourse every other day at least, from day nine or ten of the cycle for at least a week.

Effectiveness

In properly selected patients, clomiphene seems highly effective, with 70–80% of normogonadotrophic women ovulating. The pregnancy rate, however, per ovulatory cycle is 20–25%. The lower pregnancy rates could be due to coexisting tubal disease, endometriosis or male factors. The cumulative pregnancy rate over six months approaches 60–70%. Of those achieving pregnancy, half do so on the 50-mg dose, another 20% at the 100-mg dose and the rest on higher doses, with the occasional patient needing only 25 mg. The incidence of congenital anomalies is not increased, though the miscarriage rate is higher at 20–25%. This higher rate reflects the combination of better diagnosis of early pregnancy loss, the higher age in these patients and the increased incidence of multiple pregnancies.

There is evidence to suggest that cumulative pregnancy rates in women who ovulate with clomiphene and have no other infertility problems continue to rise after six cycles, but begin to plateau by about ten treatment cycles. Therefore, treatment for up to 12 cycles is recommended.

The need for monitoring with ultrasonography during clomiphene treatment may mean that GPs should prescribe the clomiphene only after the correct dose has been established at the specialist clinic. In any event, there should be a shared-care agreement between hospital and primary care.

Adverse drug reactions

Adverse reactions are not dose related and occur even with the lowest doses used. The usual adverse effects are hot flushes, in about 10% of patients, with a small minority having abdominal distension, pain, nausea, vomiting, breast tenderness, headache and hair loss (reversible). Clomiphene also has a mydriatic action and about 1.5% of patients have blurred vision and scotomas. These symptoms disappear once the drug is stopped. Significant ovarian enlargement can occur in about 5% of patients, but the full-blown OHSS is rare with clomiphene. The incidence of multiple pregnancy is about 7–10%, mostly twins. There have been higher-order pregnancies reported and in one survey 57% of triplets were due to clomiphene alone and two out of eight quadruplets and quintuplets were also due to clomiphene. This highlights the necessity for ultrasound monitoring. There is also some concern about the effects of clomiphene on oocytes and embryos. A higher incidence of neural-tube defects was noticed in one group of patients on clomiphene, but current evidence is insufficient to indicate that the causal relationship is real.

Tamoxifen

Tamoxifen is a drug similar to clomiphene with similar actions, but the trials on tamoxifen as an ovulation-induction agent are few and small in size. It appears to be as effective in inducing ovulation as clomiphene and has similar pregnancy rates.

COMBINATION OF CLOMIPHENE AND DEXAMETHASONE

Patients with high circulating levels of androgens are more resistant to clomiphene. In these patients dexamethasone 0.5 mg at night throughout the cycle is found to decrease the adrenal contribution to the circulating androgens and may result in better ovulation and conception rates.

COMBINATION OF CLOMIPHENE WITH hCG

hCG in doses of 5000–10 000 iu may be given to induce ovulation in a clomiphene treatment cycle, but the timing is important as it may not be effective if given too soon or too late. Therefore, ultrasound monitoring is needed to time the hCG when the leading follicle is of pre-ovulatory size, usually taken as at least 17 mm.

COMBINATION OF CLOMIPHENE WITH hMG

Clomiphene pre-treatment followed by daily injections of hMG has been used as a means of reducing the amount of gonadotrophins used and possibly reducing the risk of hyperstimulation and multiple gestations. There have been reports of a lower hyperstimulation rate with this regimen.

Gonadotrophins (hMG, purified FSH, recombinant FSH)

PREPARATIONS AVAILABLE

- hMG is prepared from extracts of urine from postmenopausal women. The ratio of FSH to LH is 1:1 and the commercial preparation is available with 75 iu each of FSH and LH (e.g. Pergonal®, Humegon®).
- Purified FSH (e.g. Metrodin®) consists of predominantly FSH with an FSH: LH ratio of approximately 75:1. The FSH is separated from the LH by immunochromatography.
- Recombinant FSH produced through genetic engineering has a very high purity and lacks LH. It is free of the contamination by proteins, which is seen in preparations from urinary extracts.

There is at present no evidence to suggest that purified FSH is more effective than hMG. It may be preferable to hMG in the treatment of clomiphene-resistant PCOS because of a possible decrease in moderate to severe OHSS. Similarly, recombinant FSH use has shown no significant difference in cumulative ovulation rates or pregnancy rates, or in the incidence of OHSS or multiple pregnancy as compared to purified

FSH. However, there is a reduction in the total dosage of FSH used with the recombinant FSH and the median duration of treatment is shorter.

The main indications for treatment with gonadotrophins are in WHO group I patients (low gonadotrophins and low E_2 levels) and WHO group II patients who fail to conceive with clomiphene.

METHODS OF ADMINISTRATION OF GONADOTROPHINS

hMG	Deep intramuscular injection
Purified FSH	Intramuscular or subcutaneous injection
Recombinant FSH	Subcutaneous injection

Treatment regimen

Follicular stimulation is achieved by 7–14 days of daily or alternate day hMG/FSH injections, usually beginning with 150 iu daily, starting from day two of the cycle. The patient is monitored with vaginal ultrasonography of the ovaries for the number and size of developing follicles. Periodic estimations of the circulating E_2 values may also be useful. The dose of hMG/FSH may need altering depending on the E_2 levels and the ovarian response. When scan and E_2 levels indicate that the patient is ready to receive the ovulatory stimulus (i.e. when the dominant follicle is at least 17 mm), 5000–10 000 iu hCG is given as a single injection subcutaneously. The patient is advised to have intercourse the day of the hCG injection and, if possible, for the next two days.

E_2 levels are ideally maintained below 5500 pmol/l. The risk of OHSS begins to rise from 5500–7500 pmol/l, and is significantly high over 10 000 pmol/l. Some experts, however, feel that the risk of OHSS is significantly high only with E_2 levels greater than 22 000 pmol/l. The aim of ovulation induction is to induce unifollicular ovulation with minimal occurrence of OHSS and multiple pregnancies (Figure 4.2). When E_2 levels are over 5500 pmol/l, and/or more than three follicles over 17 mm are seen, hCG should be withheld and the cycle cancelled to minimise the above-mentioned risks.

Effectiveness

Cumulative success rates of approximately 90% after six treatment cycles in WHO group I patients and 40–50% in WHO group II patients have been reported.

Adverse drug reactions

The rate of miscarriage is between 25–30%. There is no increase in congenital malformations. The risk of ectopic gestations is higher and this

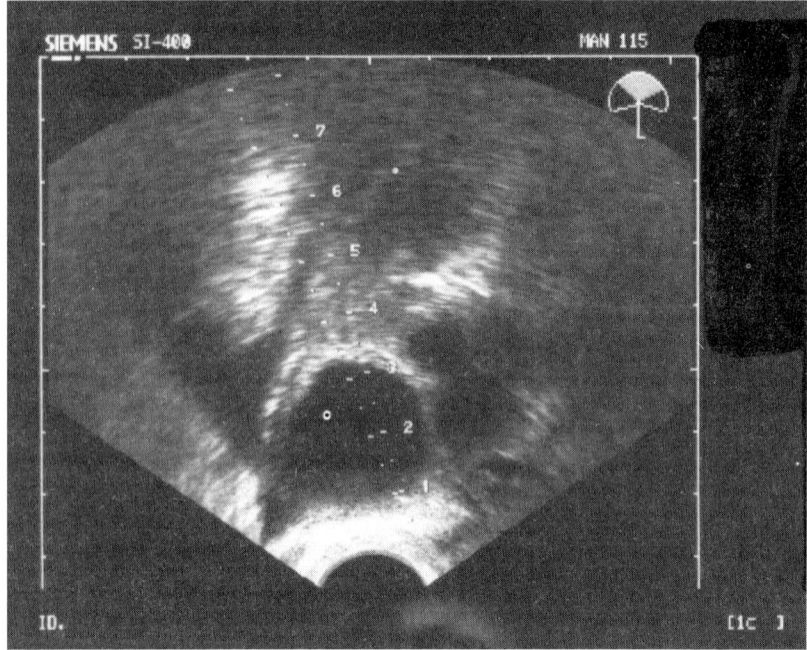

Figure 4.2   Ultrasound picture of unifollicular response to superovulation

may be due to the multiple oocytes and the high hCG levels. The rate of serious OHSS is about 1–2%. The major concern with this treatment is the high multiple-pregnancy rate of 15–20%.

LOW-DOSE GONADOTROPHIN REGIMENS

Women with polycystic ovaries are at a higher risk of developing OHSS and multiple pregnancies. The use of a low-dose step-up gonadotrophin regimen may reduce this risk. hMG/FSH is started at a dose of 75 iu daily for up to 14 days, then increased to 112.5 iu for another seven days if there is no ovarian response, then to 150 iu and so on, until the maximum dose of 225 iu daily is reached. Once ovarian activity is seen, the same dose is continued until follicular maturation is seen on ultrasonography and then the ovulatory trigger of hCG given. In 100 women treated with this protocol (Hamilton-Fairley *et al.* 1991) there was a cumulative pregnancy rate of 55% after six treatment cycles, with no case of severe OHSS. Seventy-three percent of all cycles were uniovular, with only two multiple pregnancies. The advantages of low-dose regimens are chiefly in reducing the serious risks of OHSS and multiple pregnancy in PCOS, even at the risk of lower pregnancy rates.

GONADOTROPHINS WITH GnRH AGONISTS

GnRH agonists can be used with gonadotrophins either in the long, short or ultrashort protocols. The aim of the long protocol is to conduct follicular and oocyte maturation under exogenous influences only, with no interference from possibly detrimental endogenous influences, particularly high LH levels. In patients with steady and high levels of LH, there is some evidence to suggest a higher miscarriage rate. In addition, up to 15–20% of patients may have a premature LH surge, which can result in ovulation-induction cycles being wasted. Both the short and the long protocols can prevent this from occurring. The immediate stimulatory action of GnRH agonist where it acts as the initial stimulus for follicular recruitment is made use of in the ultrashort and the short protocols.

The long protocol

The GnRH agonist is given for two to three weeks starting on day two or on day 21 of the menstrual cycle, until pituitary desensitisation is complete. An E_2 level of less than 150 pmol/l can confirm this. Follicular growth and maturation are then induced by exogenous gonadotrophins. The GnRH agonist is continued until the day of hCG administration to prevent a premature LH surge and is stopped at the same time as the hMG/FSH injections. The GnRH agonist may be in the form of a nasal spray (e.g. nafarelin) or subcutaneous injections (e.g. buserelin) in a dose of 300 to 600 mg per day. Recently, the depot GnRH injections (goserelin, e.g. Zoladex®) have been licensed for use in the long protocol for desensitisation of the pituitary.

The short and ultrashort protocols

In the short protocol, there is a one- to two-day delay between the first administration of the agonist and the gonadotrophins, and the agonist is continued until the hCG ovulatory trigger. In the ultrashort protocol there is only a brief three-day exposure of the patient to the agonist followed by gonadotrophins only.

The results from randomised studies show that there are better pregnancy rates with a larger number of oocytes and embryos obtained in patients in whom GnRH agonist has been used. This may be useful in IVF/ICSI cycles where multifollicular ovulatory response is desired (Figure 4.3), but not in superovulation cycles where, ideally, a unifollicular response is best. There has been a recent review of the literature (Hughes et al. 1998) to determine whether GnRH agonist pre-treatment in

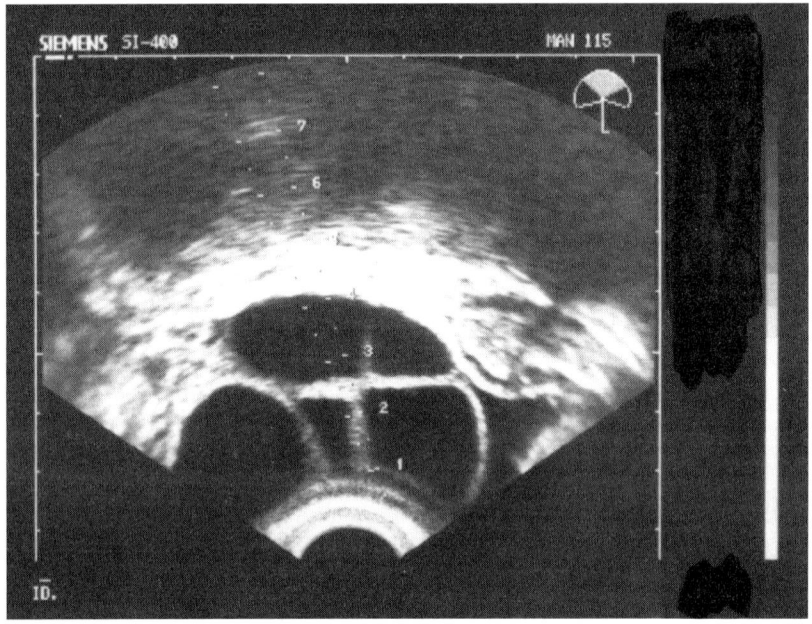

Figure 4.3 Ultrasound picture of multifollicular ovarian response in an IVF cycle

hMG/FSH cycles increases the rate of clinical pregnancy in women with PCOS, as compared to hMG/FSH alone. This showed similar pregnancy rates in the two groups, with the risks of OHSS actually being higher when GnRH agonist was used. In GnRH agonist down-regulated cycles luteal support is needed and hCG, given in the luteal phase for this purpose, increases the risk of OHSS. Therefore, there seems to be no advantage in using GnRH agonist in superovulation cycles in patients with PCOS.

Adverse drug reactions

Adverse effects of the GnRH agonists include menopausal symptoms, but these are not common as the patient is on the drug for only a short period of time.

GONADOTROPHINS WITH GnRH ANTAGONISTS (CETRORELIX, GANIRELIX)

GnRH antagonists, which allow suppression of LH surges, have recently become available and are being evaluated. In comparison to GnRH agonists, which require a long period of administration to achieve down-regulation of receptors and desensitisation of the gonadotrophic cells, GnRH antagonists bind competitively to the receptors and thereby prevent the endogenous GnRH from exerting its stimulatory effects on the pituitary cells. Within hours the secretion of gonadotrophins is reduced. This allows for more flexible and shorter protocols.

PULSATILE ADMINISTRATION OF GnRH AGONISTS

GnRH agonists, when administered continuously, result in pituitary desensitisation and down regulation with a reduction in FSH and LH values. But when administered in a pulsatile fashion, which mimics normal secretion, it can lead to increased gonadotrophin secretion.

Indications for use

The use of GnRH agonists in a pulsatile manner is mainly indicated in women with hypogonadotrophic hypogonadism (WHO group I), where endogenous GnRH is dysfunctional or absent. One example is anovulation associated with weight loss where there are low FSH and E_2 levels, but here treatment should be deferred until the BMI is over 20 kg/m², for reasons referred to later in this chapter. This treatment may also have a role in clomiphene-resistant WHO group II patients, but a patient who is obese with hyperandrogenic PCOS and high circulating levels of LH does not do well on this regimen. Pulsatile GnRH agonists may also be useful in a patient who is hyperprolactinaemic and cannot tolerate bromocriptine/cabergoline.

Method of administration

The GnRH agonist is administered subcutaneously or intravenously through a pump that must be worn continuously. The reconstituted GnRH agonist is stable for about three weeks and is administered in pulses of 15 to 20 mg boluses for the subcutaneous dose and 5 µg boluses for the intravenous route every 60–120 minutes, usually every 90 minutes. This dose may be increased by 5 µg every week if there is no response. The patient is monitored with periodic E_2 levels and ultrasonography to detect follicular growth. Usually ovulation occurs around day 14 and the couple are advised to have intercourse at around that time. The luteal phase is maintained by either continuing the pump, with hCG injections or progestogen pessaries.

Effectiveness

The cumulative pregnancy rates in patients with hypothalamic amenorrhoea at the end of 12 cycles is around 80–90% with a 20–30% pregnancy rate per treatment cycle. In patients with PCOS the cumulative pregnancy rate is about 30%. The miscarriage rate is around 20% and there is no increase in the incidence of congenital anomalies. The advantage of GnRH agonist use is the reduced number of multiple pregnancies (about 4–5%) as compared to other ovulation-induction methods as the feedback system is intact. The risk of OHSS is also low and that of severe OHSS is almost nil. The problems of this regimen are more to do with the local reactions and infections at the site of needle placement or technical problems with the pump. Evidence suggests that this treatment is effective and safe in properly selected patients (Balen *et al.* 1994; Martin *et al.* 1993). However, it is not widely used and has gained little patient acceptance in view of the inconvenience of wearing the pump continuously, the need for the injection site to be changed from time to time and the expense of the pumps.

KEYPOINTS

- Ovulation induction should be performed only after male and tubal factors have been ruled out.
- Clomiphene is the most commonly prescribed drug for ovulation induction.
- It is necessary to monitor at least the first clomiphene cycle with ultrasonography due to the risk of multiple pregnancy and the variable response of patients to different doses of clomiphene.
- The major concern with gonadotrophin treatment is the high multiple pregnancy rate.
- Women with polycystic ovaries are at a higher risk of developing OHSS and multiple pregnancies. The use of a low-dose step-up gonadotrophin regimen may reduce this risk.
- GnRH is the treatment of choice in patients with hypogonadotrophic hypogonadism.
- The advantages of GnRH-agonist treatment are the reduced number of multiple pregnancies and low risk of OHSS compared to the other ovulation induction methods.

Iatrogenic problems of ovulation induction

OVARIAN HYPERSTIMULATION SYNDROME

OHSS is a potentially life-threatening adverse effect of ovulation induction. It is rarely seen with anti-oestrogens occurring mainly with the use of gonadotrophins, especially when GnRH agonist analogues are used in combination. To occur it needs luteinisation by hCG (given as an ovulatory trigger, as luteal support, when pregnancy occurs or by endogenous LH). The quoted incidence of OHSS occurring in ovulation induction cycles is 0.25–0.9%. In IVF/ICSI cycles, where GnRH agonist is used with gonadotrophins, the incidence may be 6–14%.

The basic pathology is a shift of fluid from the intravascular to the extravascular space. The increased vascular permeability allowing this shift is thought to be due to various agents including LH, histamine, prostaglandins and prorenins from the ovaries and, in recent times, vascular endothelial growth factor.

The clinical symptomatology includes cystic ovarian enlargement with ascites, pleural effusion and rarely pericardial effusion. The intravascular volume depletion leads to:

- dehydration
- hypovolaemia
- electrolyte disturbances
- thrombosis due to the haemoconcentration.

OHSS is usually classified according to its severity (Table 4.2).

Risk factors for OHSS

Although any woman undergoing ovarian stimulation is at risk of OHSS, some women seem to be more at risk (Table 4.3).

Prevention of OHSS

The prevention of OHSS depends primarily on carrying out ovulation induction only in centres with appropriate monitoring for serum E_2 and

Table 4.2 Classification of ovarian hyperstimulation syndrome (adapted from RCOG Guidelines No. 5, 1995)

Severity	Clinical features	Ultrasound findings
Mild	Abdominal bloating with some pain	Ovaries < than 8 cm
Moderate	Nausea, vomiting and increased abdominal discomfort	Ovaries 8–12 cm Evidence of ascites
Severe	May be critically ill with clinical ascites ± hydrothorax with hypovolaemia and oliguria May have thromboembolic problems due to haemoconcentration In critically ill patients adult respiratory distress syndrome may be seen Biochemical features of haemoconcentration, renal + liver dysfunction	Ovaries > 12 cm Ascites

Table 4.3	Risk factors for OHSS

- Women under 35 years

- Low BMI

- PCOS

- Use of GnRH agonists in combination with gonadotrophins

- Use of exogenous hCG either as ovulatory trigger or luteal support

- Endogenous surge of hCG due to pregnancy

- Many small and intermediate follicles (< 14 mm)

- High E_2 level (>10 000 pmol/l)

- Large number oocytes (> 20) collected in IVF/ICSI cycles

ultrasonography. Consideration should be given to those methods of ovulation induction with the lowest incidence of OHSS. These include the low-dose step-up regimen rather than the GnRH agonist and hMG/FSH combination cycles, using pulsatile GnRH where appropriate and a laparoscopic ovarian drilling in patients with PCOS.

If E_2 levels are excessively high or many follicles appear while monitoring ovarian stimulation, serious consideration should be given to the cancellation of cycles. The ovulatory trigger of hCG can be withheld, although this does not totally remove the risk of OHSS as the spontaneous LH surge may still occur in non-GnRH agonist cycles. If oocyte recovery has taken place in ART cycles, and an increased number of oocytes obtained, then the embryo transfer may be deferred to prevent a conception cycle and the embryos cryopreserved to be used at a later date. Luteal-phase support with progesterone rather than hCG may reduce the risk in high-risk women.

Prophylactic intravenous albumin administration at around the time of oocyte recovery has been used as a method of preventing OHSS in a high-risk patient, but its usefulness in this situation needs further validation.

Treatment of OHSS

This is mainly supportive. OHSS undergoes gradual resolution with time (in non-pregnant patients in about seven days; in pregnant patients about 10–20 days). There is no increase in miscarriage rates in conception cycles with OHSS.

Analgesics such as paracetamol, codeine and opiates and anti-emetics can be used for the relief of discomfort and gastrointestinal symptoms. Oral fluid replacement to counter the haemoconcentration may be given in mild/moderate cases or, if the patient cannot tolerate this, intravenous crystalloids may be administered. In more severe cases with significant hypovolaemia or ascites, albumin is the volume expander of choice, as crystalloids may actually worsen the ascites – 500 ml of 4.5% isotonic albumin can be given intravenously within two hours quite safely in a healthy young adult, but close monitoring of the haemodynamic status would be needed when larger volumes are required in severe hypovolaemia. Ultrasound-guided paracentesis, to avoid enlarged ovaries, may be required to relieve severe pulmonary compromise or relieve pressure on the renal veins and inferior vena cava. Pressure on the latter reduces venous return to the heart, worsening the hypovolaemia and renal perfusion. Antidiuretics should be avoided. Compression stockings, ambulation and correction of haemoconcentration are used to prevent thromboembolism and prophylactic anticoagulant therapy should be considered in severe cases. Surgery is only undertaken if there is torsion of the ovaries or rupture leading to haemorrhage. Ovaries are friable and easily traumatised and surgery should be avoided unless indicated by the clinical situation.

MULTIPLE PREGNANCY

The risks of multiple pregnancy with ovulation induction vary from 7–10% for clomiphene to 15–20% with gonadotrophins. Two or, at most, three embryos are replaced in the uterus with ART cycles, so more triplets, quadruplets and higher-order pregnancies follow ovulation induction rather than IVF/ICSI cycles. In one survey (Levene *et al.* 1992), 52% of higher-order pregnancies (excluding twins) were conceived after clomiphene treatment and 33% after gonadotrophin treatment.

The risks of multiple pregnancy increase exponentially with every baby, for both the mother and the babies. Apart from problems for the mother, which include an increased incidence of pre-eclampsia, antepartum and postpartum haemorrhage, there are also the emotional, financial and physical burdens on the parents of bringing up the children. Prematurity is the most important reason for the increase in perinatal morbidity and mortality, compounded by possible associated growth restriction. Twins are four times and triplets five times as likely to be stillborn as compared to singletons, and have a perinatal morbidity rate that is five times and eight times higher than for singletons, respectively. The cerebral palsy rate among singletons is around 1.6 per 1000 live births, while for twins it is 7.4 and for triplets 26.7 per 1000 live births.

The close monitoring of patients during ovulation induction and strict criteria for the cancellation of cycles or conversion to IVF are extremely important in preventing the problems of multiple birth. In addition, it is important to counsel patients and to discuss the possibility of fetal reduction in higher-order pregnancies, an ethically contentious issue. While fetal reduction in quadruplets and higher-order pregnancies may benefit the remaining fetuses, its use in triplet pregnancies remains contentious; there is a miscarriage rate of 12–13% following fetal reduction as compared to 6% with unreduced triplet pregnancies.

THE ASSOCIATION OF OVARIAN CARCINOMA WITH OVULATION INDUCTION

A number of recent reports have indicated a higher than expected rate of ovarian cancer in women having drug treatment for infertility. Concerns have been raised about the exposure of the ovaries to supraphysiological levels of gonadotrophins, the occurrence of multiple ovulations and trauma to the epithelial surface resulting from treatment with clomiphene and gonadotrophins. But before any risk is attributed to the drugs alone, the association between parity, infertility and ovarian malignancies has to be considered. Nulliparous women without any interventions for infertility have almost double the risk of ovarian carcinoma as compared to parous women. Conversely, infertile women with or without treatment who later go on to give birth have the same risk as any other parous woman. Though there is a clear-cut association between parity and ovarian carcinoma, the available evidence does not lead to a firm link between ovulation-induction agents and ovarian cancer. The risk, if it does exist, has been estimated at an annual increase of less than one in 5000. Such a risk would have to be balanced against the potential benefits of a pregnancy.

At present, it is thought that clomiphene is not associated with any increased risk of ovarian cancer when used for less than 12 cycles. Until

---

KEYPOINTS
- Before embarking on ovulation induction, it is essential to counsel patients regarding the risks of OHSS, multiple pregnancy and the possibility of fetal reduction, and the putative risks of cancer of the ovary.
- More triplets/quadruplets and higher order pregnancies follow ovulation induction rather than IVF/ICSI cycles.
- The risks of multiple pregnancy increase exponentially with every baby, for both the mother and the babies.
- There should be guidelines within every unit on reducing the risks of OHSS and multiple pregnancy, and those treatment regimens that reduce these risks.

there are more data from large-scale epidemiological studies, it would seem prudent to use gonadotrophins for the least number of cycles and at the lowest effective doses possible. Before embarking on any treatment for ovulation induction, a full discussion with the patients of the risk-benefit analysis on the current treatment available with regard to cancer of the ovary is advisable.

Hyperprolactinaemia

Prolactin is a protein hormone secreted by the anterior pituitary. Raised levels of prolactin interfere with the pulsatile release of GnRH from the hypothalamus. This in turn may cause amenorrhoea, oligomenorrhoea, anovulation and subfertility. There may be associated galactorrhoea in 30–80% of cases.

AETIOLOGY

High prolactin levels may be due to increased secretion from the anterior pituitary due to micro- and macroadenomas, or due to the inhibition of the action of dopamine, which is the main inhibitory regulator of prolactin (PIF – prolactin inhibitory factor). Drugs such as phenothiazines and other antipsychotics may have this inhibitory effect. Approximately 50% of patients with hyperprolactinaemia show evidence of pituitary microadenomas; macroadenomas are rare and 30% of cases are idiopathic. Other causes include:

- drugs
- stress
- renal or hepatic dysfunction
- hypothyroidism.

In the latter case the increased TRH acts as a stimulator of prolactin secretion. Around 9% of patients with PCOS may have increased prolactin levels but the pathophysiology of this is not clear. There are different theories, one of which suggests that the raised unopposed E_2 levels in PCOS may directly stimulate the secretion of prolactin from the anterior pituitary, and another which suggests that the hyperprolactinaemia itself may stimulate adrenal and ovarian androgen biosynthesis, hence causing PCOS.

TREATMENT OPTIONS

Patients with macroadenomas need treatment irrespective of the severity of symptoms or the need for fertility, due to the risks of tumour expansion. Patients with hyperprolactinaemia without evidence of a macroadenoma also need to be treated, as they are hypo-oestrogenic and need oestrogen to maintain skeletal integrity.

Surgery is usually indicated only in patients with nonsecretory pituitary adenomas or parasellar tumours who, despite normalisation of prolactin levels and possible improvement in visual fields, do not show considerable tumour shrinkage, or in patients with large macroadenomas intolerant or resistant to drug treatment. Surgery results in long-term normalisation of prolactin values only in about 50% of microadenomas and 10–15% of macroadenomas.

However, surgery is infrequently employed as good results are obtained with medical therapy and this forms the most effective and main line of treatment for hyperprolactinaemia. The most tried and tested dopamine agonist is bromocriptine.

Bromocriptine

This is a semisynthetic ergot alkaloid and has been in use since 1971. It is effective in shrinking 80% of macroadenomas in over 80–90% of patients, whose prolactin levels return to normal. It also stops galactorrhoea and restores ovulation in 70–80% of patients. Problems with bromocriptine include its short half-life, which necessitates treatment two or three times daily. Adverse effects are common and are mostly seen at the start of treatment. These include nausea, headache, vertigo, postural hypotension, fatigue and drowsiness. About 5% of patients need to stop treatment because of intolerable adverse effects. They can be minimised by initiating treatment with a low dose of bromocriptine (1.25 mg) at bedtime with a snack, to be gradually increased up to 2.5 mg three times a day with food over two to three weeks. Administration by a vaginal pessary, a depot injection monthly and a slow release oral preparation have also been used.

Cabergoline

Cabergoline is a newer dopamine agonist recently licensed for treatment of hyperprolactinaemia. It is rapidly becoming the treatment of choice for most patients because of its many benefits over bromocriptine. These include a longer half-life, which simplifies administration at 0.5–1 mg twice weekly. There are significantly fewer adverse effects, especially with regard to the gastrointestinal tract. Two large randomised controlled trials have shown cabergoline to be more effective than bromocriptine in restoring normoprolactinaemia and ovulation, with fewer adverse effects (Webster *et al*. 1994; Pascal *et al*. 1995).

Quinogolide

Quinogolide is another new dopamine agonist found to be as effective as bromocriptine, but when compared to cabergoline adverse effects were fewer with the latter. It is more expensive and is worth considering only in women resistant to bromocriptine or cabergoline.

Problems associated with pregnancy

None of these drugs has been associated with increased rates of miscarriage, congenital anomalies or any other problems associated with pregnancy, but the current practice is to stop the drug if pregnancy occurs. This may be unnecessary with bromocriptine particularly if there is evidence of a prolactinoma, which may enlarge in pregnancy. Data are too few as yet regarding cabergoline.

KEYPOINTS
- Medical therapy forms the most effective and main line of treatment of hyperprolactinaemia. The most tried and tested dopamine agonist is bromocriptine.
- Cabergoline is rapidly becoming the drug of choice in treating hyperprolactinaemia.

Other treatment modalities for oligo/anovulation

DIETARY/PSYCHOTHERAPY

Patients with weight loss or hypothalamic oligo/amenorrhoea

In this group of patients, weight gain resulting in a BMI of over 20 kg/m^2 is the most effective treatment, though this can be difficult to achieve. It is important to resist the temptation of inducing ovulation in the underweight patient using pulsatile GnRH, though this may be successful. Underweight women are significantly more at risk of anaemia and preterm labour and of having babies with low birth weight, or growth restriction. Some women may have difficulty in caring for their offspring if they have psychological problems. Therefore, treatment should be deferred until dietary and psychotherapy support is provided to achieve a BMI of over 20 kg/m^2.

Patients with obesity (BMI of over 30 kg/m^2)

A supervised weight loss programme is advised for any woman with a BMI of over 30 kg/m^2, whether ovulatory or not. This is a Grade A recommendation based on evidence from a randomised controlled trial. Weight loss increases ovulation and pregnancy rates both spontaneously as well as with ovulation induction regimens and reduces other problems associated with obesity. Accurate recording of BMI at the first visit, with a weight loss programme for six months, is a first-line management for the treatment of subfertility in obese patients.

LAPAROSCOPIC DRILLING OF THE OVARIES

Current evidence suggests that laparoscopic drilling of the ovaries by laser or diathermy is as effective as gonadotrophins in inducing ovulation in women with anovulatory PCOS, resistant to treatment with clomiphene (Farquhar *et al*. 1998). One RCT compared ovarian diathermy, followed by clomiphene only if spontaneous menstruation failed to occur, with hMG. There was no significant difference in the percentage of women who ovulated, the cumulative pregnancy rate after six cycles and the live-birth rate.

The advantages of ovarian diathermy include a lower incidence of multiple gestation and the absence of hyperstimulation. Laparoscopic ovarian drilling may also be beneficial in increasing ovarian sensitivity to subsequent clomiphene and gonadotrophins, even if spontaneous ovulation does not result from the surgery.

The risks associated with this treatment are mainly operative, including diathermy or laser damage. The reported incidence of post-treatment adhesions varies widely and lysis of these laparoscopically three to four weeks after the initial treatment does not improve pregnancy rates. The long-term problems of premature menopause are still being evaluated but, so far, in women followed up for about ten years there is no evidence of an increased risk. Therefore, it seems that laparoscopic ovarian drilling by laser or diathermy should be considered as an alternative to gonadotrophin treatment in women with PCOS who fail to ovulate with clomiphene.

EGG DONATION

This is discussed in greater detail in Chapter 8; it may be the only option open for patients with ovarian failure. Such patients should also be offered HRT because of the long-term problems of osteoporosis and cardiovascular disease.

KEYPOINTS
- The BMI in patients undergoing ovulation induction should ideally be between 20–30 kg/m^2.
- Laparoscopic ovarian drilling should be considered as an alternative to gonadotrophin treatment in women with PCOS who fail to ovulate with clomiphene.

Conclusions

In conclusion, the treatment of anovulatory infertility with the current available regimens can be successful in many cases, but it is not without risk. Relevant investigation and appropriate treatment is necessary. Ovulation induction should be performed only in centres with adequate monitoring facilities and there should be clear guidelines and protocols for reducing the risks of OHSS and multiple gestation.

References

Balen, A.H., Bratt, D.D., West, C., Patel, A. and Jacobs, H.S. (1994) Cumulative conception and live birth rates after the treatment of anovulatory infertility: safety and efficacy of ovulation induction in 200 patients. *Hum Reprod* **9**, 1563–70

Farquhar, C., Vandekerckhove, P., Amot, M. and Lilford, R. (1998) Polycystic ovary syndrome: laparoscopic 'drilling' by diathermy or laser for ovulation induction in patients with anovulatory polycystic ovarian syndrome (Cochrane Review). *The Cochrane Library*, Issue 3. Oxford: Update Software

Hamilton-Fairley, D., Kiddy, D., Watson, L., Sagle, M. and Franks, S. (1991) Low-dose gonadotrophin therapy for induction of ovulation in 100 women with polycystic ovary syndrome. *Hum Reprod* **6**, 1095–99

Hughes, E., Collins, J. and Vandekerckhove, P. (1998) Gonadotrophin releasing hormone analogue as an adjunct to gonadotrophin therapy for clomiphene-resistant PCOS (Cochrane Review). *The Cochrane Library*, Issue 2. Oxford: Update Software

Levene, M.I., Wild, J. and Steer, P. (1992) Higher multiple births and the modern management of infertility in Britain. *Br J Obstet Gynaecol* **99**, 607–13

Martin, K.A., Hall, J.E., Adams, J.M. and Crowley, W.F. Jr (1993) Comparisons of exogenous gonadotrophins and pulsatile gonadotrophin-releasing hormone for induction of ovulation in hypogonadotrophic amenorrhoea. *J Clin Endocrinol Metab* **77**, 125–9

Pascal Vigneron, V., Weyha, G., Bosc, M. and Leclere, J. (1995) Hyperprolactinaemic amenorrhoea: treatment with cabergoline versus bromocriptine. Results of a national multicentre randomised double blind study. *Presse Medicale* **24**, 753–7

Royal College of Obstetricians and Gynaecologists (1995) *Management and Prevention of Ovarian Hyperstimulation Syndrome (OHSS)*. London: RCOG (RCOG Guidelines, No. 5)

Webster, J., Piscitelli, G., Polli, A., Ferrari, C.I., Ismail, I. and Scanlon, M.F. (1994) A comparison of cabergoline and bromocriptine in the treatment of hyperprolactinaemic amenorrhoea. *N Engl J Med* **331**, 904–9

5 Tubal-factor infertility

Introduction

The fallopian tube plays an essential role in the process of conception, being necessary for egg pick-up, fertilisation and embryo transport. Egg pick-up is dependent upon the action of the tubal fimbriae guiding the ovulated egg into the tube. Egg and embryo transport results from the unidirectional beating of the tubal cilia coupled with peristaltic contractions of the muscular tubal wall. Secretions from the tubal epithelium nourish the embryo.

Tubal-factor infertility includes an array of disorders affecting one or more of the above components, in the form of peritubal adhesions, proximal and/or distal tubal blockage and hydrosalpinx formation (Figure 5.1). Even in the presence of a patent tube, damage to the inner tubal structures may result in severe impairment of tubal function.

Tubal disease is one of the major causes of female infertility, affecting between 10% and 30% of infertile couples. It plays a particularly important role in secondary infertility, accounting for approximately 40% of cases. It is also probably the only major preventable cause of infertility.

Aetiology

Tubal-factor infertility can result from a variety of causes including infection, surgery, congenital abnormalities and endometriosis.

INFECTION

The major cause of tubal-factor infertility is pelvic inflammatory disease (PID). Cohort studies involving over 1000 women with laparoscopically confirmed PID found at least a 10% risk of tubal-factor infertility following an episode of PID. The risk increased considerably with further infections (Table 5.1).

Most cases of PID follow an episode of sexually transmitted disease (STD) due to either *Chlamydia trachomatis* or *Neisseria gonorrhoeae*. Of these,

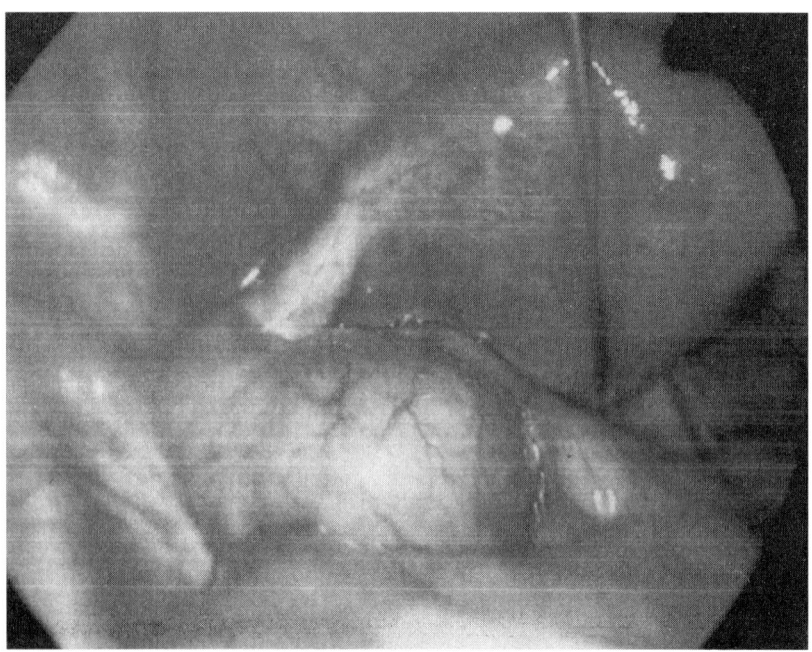

Figure 5.1 Diagnostic laparoscopy showing the uterus and right hydrosalpinx

chlamydia is the most important. This is now the most common STD in the UK and Europe and is recognised as being responsible for at least 50% of identifiable cases of PID. The risks of acquiring both chlamydia and PID are age-related, with women under 25 years of age at highest risk. Rates of chlamydial infection and PID continue to rise, accelerated by chlamydia's asymptomatic nature. It is not surprising, therefore, that the majority of women with tubal-factor infertility give no history of chlamydia or PID, and that three-quarters of women with tubal-factor infertility have chlamydial antibodies compared with only one quarter of controls. PID can be prevented by screening for chlamydia infection (Scholes *et al.* 1996).

Table 5.1 Increasing risk of tubal-factor infertility (TFI)

Episodes of PID (n)	Risk of TFI
1	13%
2	35%
3 or more	75%

Gonorrhoea, on the other hand, has a more symptomatic clinical course, but has declined in incidence dramatically compared to chlamydia. In a recent multicentre trial screening abortion patients (Penney *et al.* 1998) chlamydia was found to be almost 30 times more common than gonorrhoea. Other organisms which play a lesser role include:

- anaerobic and haemolytic streptococci
- staphylococcus
- bacteroides
- *Escherichia coli*
- mycoplasma species
- *Clostridium welchii*
- actinomyces
- tuberculosis.

The latter must be borne in mind, however, if the woman is a recent immigrant from an at-risk area. The anaerobic commensals are usually seen in older women or in cases of tubo-ovarian abscess. The contribution of bacterial vaginosis remains uncertain.

PID may occur subclinically or may complicate:

- miscarriage
- the puerperium
- intrauterine instrumentation
- lower abdominal and pelvic surgery.

SURGERY

Lower abdominal surgery is a risk factor for tubal-factor infertility. Most abdominal and pelvic surgery causes adhesions. Gynaecological operations carry a recognisable risk due to the proximity of the operating field to the fallopian tubes. More recently, the role of uterine instrumentation has been highlighted. Procedures such as IUCD insertion and surgical evacuation of the uterus may facilitate the dissemination of endocervical chlamydia to the upper genital tract. The risk is thought to be approximately 14% and is likely to account for the increased proportion of tubal-factor infertility in cases of secondary infertility.

A history of abdominal operations such as appendicectomy, bowel resection and major urological procedures also identifies those who need early tubal evaluation in their infertility investigation schedule.

OTHER CAUSES

Congenital abnormalities are uncommon, and may be associated with developmental anomalies of the urinary system. Ultrasonic or in some cases radiological assessment of the woman's urinary system is therefore recommended. Moderate or severe endometriosis can cause anatomical distortion to the tubo-ovarian relationship. Intraluminal endometriosis is a recognised but rare cause of tubal blockage. Endometriosis is further discussed in Chapter 6.

Pathology

ACUTE INFLAMMATION

The inflammatory changes of endosalpingitis follow acute endometritis with spread to the mucosa of the fallopian tube, damaging the cilia and epithelial cells. The inflammation of interstitial salpingitis involves the whole wall of the tube, including the mesosalpinx, and results in swelling of the tubal wall.

CHRONIC INFLAMMATION

Intraluminal adhesions lead to partial obstruction and the risk of ectopic pregnancy or complete obstruction and tubal-factor infertility. Extraluminal adhesions form secondary to salpingo-oophoritis. A pyosalpinx may form and progress to peritonitis or the inflammation may subside with development of a hydrosalpinx. The condition of chronic PID is characterised by persistent pelvic pain and/or dyspareunia. It is unclear whether the symptoms are secondary to the associated adhesions or due to continuing low-grade infection.

Tubal classification

Unlike the accepted scoring system for pelvic endometriosis established by the American Fertility Society, several scoring systems for tubal damage have been developed but none has gained universal acceptance. The aim of such a classification would be to predict those women who would benefit most from surgery, to quantify the prognosis and allow objective comparison of different surgical techniques and operators.

The best-known grading system assesses the degree of adhesions, salpingitis and tubal occlusion (Wu and Gocial 1988). The degree of pathology is subjectively scored into four grades:

- mild
- moderate
- severe
- extensive.

There is a significant correlation between score and cumulative pregnancy rates. Surgery for milder disease is more likely to lead to acceptable two-year pregnancy rates of around 50%, but surgery for severe or extensive disease is unlikely to be beneficial. Adequate tubal assessment is therefore essential prior to embarking on surgery.

KEYPOINTS
- The major cause of tubal-factor infertility is pelvic inflammatory disease.
- *Chlamydia trachomatis* is the organism responsible for most cases of PID.
- Rates of PID can be reduced by screening for chlamydia.
- Adequate tubal assessment is essential prior to embarking on surgery.

Treatment

CONSERVATIVE

Figure 5.2 shows the cumulative conception rates with untreated tubal disease compared with fertile couples. Up to 10% of the pregnancies are ectopic. Fecundity is much reduced in the tubal group, with the majority of pregnancies occurring in the first 12 months of diagnosis.

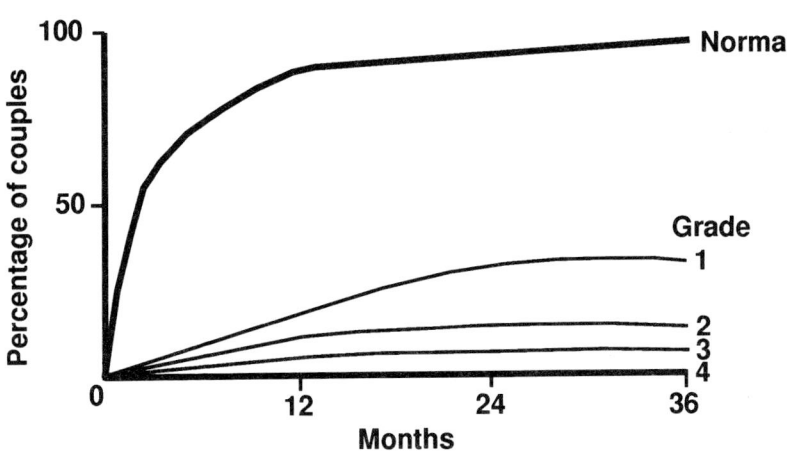

Figure 5.2 Cumulative conception rates related to disease grading, compared with normal (adapted from Wu and Gocial 1988)

MEDICAL

The role of antibiotic therapy in cases of tubal-factor infertility secondary to PID is unproven. In general, however, tertiary prevention fails because substantial tubal damage has already occurred by the time the patient presents with tubal-factor infertility. Women with tuberculosis require chemotherapy, but this will not repair the damage present.

FACTORS TO BE TAKEN INTO ACCOUNT BEFORE DECIDING ON SURGERY

Female age	Each year after 40 years of age, fecundity dramatically decreases. If ovarian function is normal, treatment decisions should reflect a careful analysis of chances of success balanced against the risks involved.
Cause of tubal disease	In cases of tubal-factor infertility due to tuberculosis, for example, medical management, followed by IVF, is most appropriate.
Extent of tubal disease	In general, the more severe the tubal disease, the lower the pregnancy rate and the higher the ectopic rate when managed by surgery.
Previous surgical treatment	A patient with a history of ectopic pregnancy has a significant risk (approximately 15%) of recurrence.
Presence of other infertility factors	These may identify those who would most benefit from assisted reproduction.
Surgical experience and appropriate facilities	Tubal surgery should only be carried out by operators who have had the appropriate training and in centres where there are appropriate facilities and trained staff, with sufficient patient throughput to maintain experience.
Financial	The cost of privately funded treatment may be beyond the couple's means.

In general, surgery offers the best results when carried out in properly selected women

---

SURGERY

Surgery has an important complementary role to IVF in the management of patients with tubal-factor infertility. Counselling is complex and many factors must be taken into account before a decision on surgery is made.

Surgical options

The main advantage of surgery is that the chance of success is continuous, at least in the first one to two years following surgery. However, this needs to be weighed against an increased risk of ectopic pregnancy.

PROXIMAL TUBAL OBSTRUCTION

Proximal tubal obstruction may occur in both the intramural segment or at the uterotubal junction and accounts for 10–25% of tubal-factor infertility. Causes include:

- obliterative fibrosis
- salpingitis isthmica nodosa
- congenital abnormalities
- polyps
- intramucosal endometriosis
- chronic inflammation.

However, up to 40% of women will have no permanent obstruction despite having a positive laparoscopy or hysterosalpingogram. Apparent blocks are usually a result of tubal spasm or transient occlusion by mucous plugs.

Diagnostic selective salpingography (DSS) is the best method for differentiating true proximal tubal obstruction from spurious blocks due to spasm or plugs. It also delineates the exact site or sites of occlusion. The only contraindications to the procedure include:

- pregnancy
- active pelvic infection
- allergy to iodinated contrast media.

Complications are few but include minor pelvic pain and vaginal spotting. The radiation dose is equivalent to that of a barium enema.

Under antibiotic cover, the patient is placed in modified lithotomy position on a screening table. The perineum is cleansed and draped and a speculum inserted. Following cleaning of the cervix, a local anaesthetic spray is used. Intravenous sedation may be used as an alternative. A preliminary hysterosalpingogram is usually undertaken (Figure 5.3). Under screening control, DSS is performed by advancing a curved

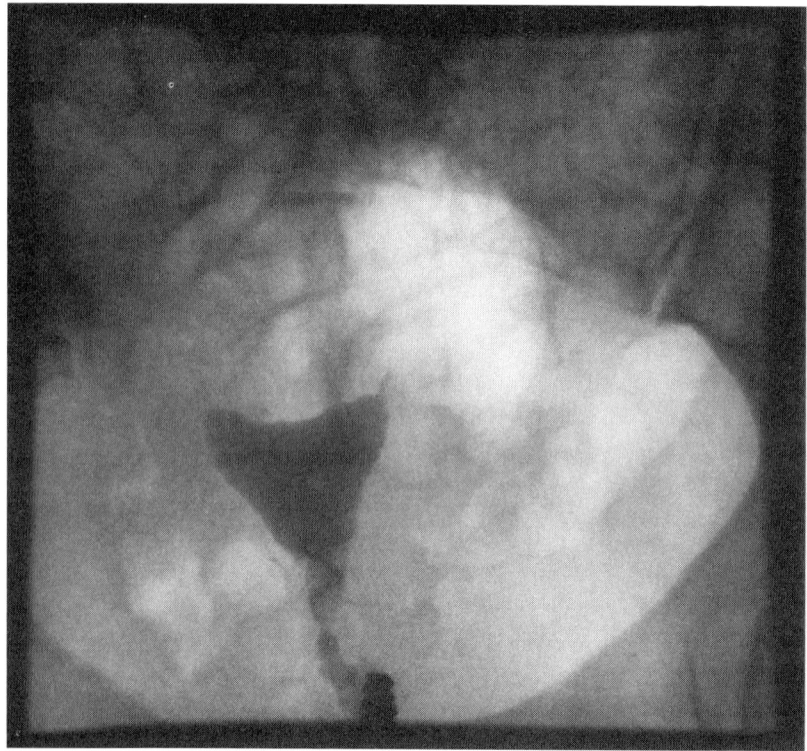

Figure 5.3   Hysterosalpingogram showing bilateral proximal tubal obstruction

catheter into the tubal ostium. The cannula is abutted against the intrauterine ostia and radio-opaque medium is injected into the fallopian tube. This confirms whether proximal tubal obstruction is present.

Tubal catheterisation is always preceded by DSS, although both procedures are usually performed in the same session. Radiological, falloposcopic, hysteroscopic and ultrasound imaging of a variety of catheters, guide-wires and balloon systems can be used to attempt recanalisation of the proximally obstructed fallopian tubes (Figure 5.4). These different methods have not been compared, so it is not possible to recommend one over another. The procedure takes approximately 30 minutes and offers outpatient diagnosis and treatment in one session that can be repeated (Figure 5.5). It is only available in specialist centres.

No prospective studies have been controlled so it is difficult to comment on the resulting pregnancy rates. A review of 11 studies (479

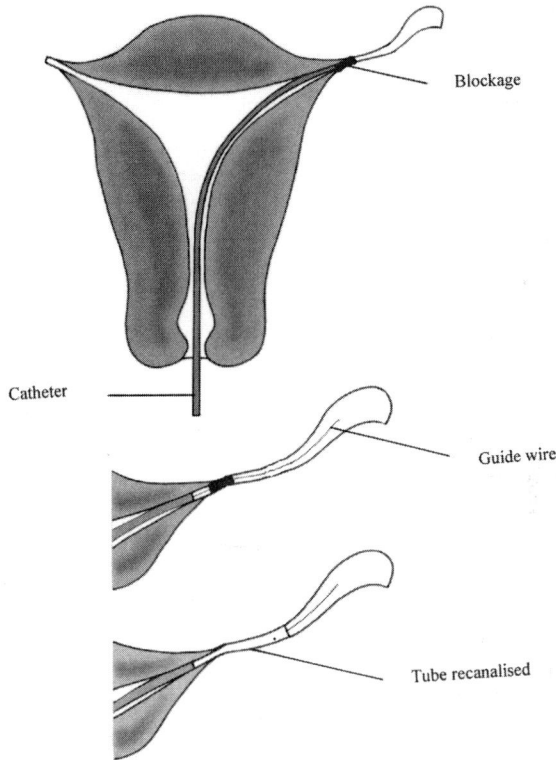

Figure 5.4 Tubal catheterisation

patients) found an 82% patency rate with a 24% pregnancy rate, of which 3% were ectopic pregnancies (Thurmond 1994). The RCOG and American Fertility Society now recommend that tubal catheterisation be attempted before tubal microsurgery or IVF in patients with proximal tubal obstruction.

Surgical management also involves tubocornual anastomosis and segmental resection, which carries a recognised risk of pregnancy-related uterine rupture if the procedure has involved cutting into the myometrium.

There are no RCTs or controlled studies that compare tubal surgery with tubal catheterisation for proximal tubal obstruction. In the case of tubocornual anastomosis, however, success rates are limited with two studies finding a monthly fecundity of 3.5% (Jacobs *et al.* 1988; Gillett and Herbison 1989). Microsurgical techniques have not been shown to offer any significant advantage over conventional surgery.

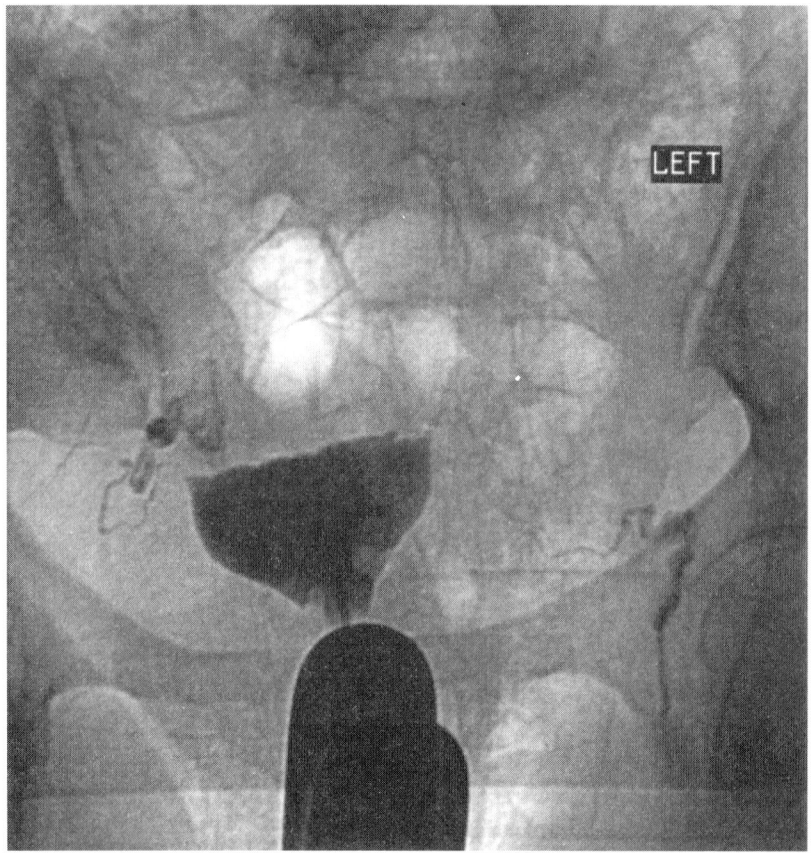

Figure 5.5   Bilateral tubal patency following tubal catheterisation

DISTAL TUBAL OBSTRUCTION

Adhesiolysis

Adhesiolysis appears to confer some benefit over no treatment and can result in cumulative intrauterine pregnancy rates of 60% at two years. However, patients with thicker, vascular or extensive adhesions have a much poorer prognosis, with a cumulative two-year pregnancy rate of around 13%. Various methods exist:

- laparotomy with lysis performed microscopically
- laparotomy with lysis performed macroscopically
- laparoscopically using blunt/sharp dissection, electrocautery or CO_2 laser.

At present, no single technique appears to be superior in preventing adhesion reformation or improving pregnancy rates. The issue of whether laparoscopy is better than laparotomy remains unclear as no prospective randomised controlled trials have been carried out. The RCOG suggests that a laparoscopic approach can be used for adhesiolysis, with recognition that the technique results in a shorter hospital stay and an earlier return to activities.

With regard to the surgical technique, a meta-analysis of a number of non-randomised controlled trials revealed a statistically significant increase in the pregnancy rate and decrease in ectopic pregnancy rates with microsurgery.

Salpingostomy

Distal tubal occlusion, with varying degrees of dilatation of the distal tube, is most commonly the result of PID. Tubal function is generally severely compromised.

In general, pregnancy outcome is directly correlated to the tubal disease score. Salpingostomy for minimal to mild tubal damage (stage 1–2) produces three times the pregnancy rates of moderate to severe disease. Surgical expertise is essential. Surgery performed by a general gynaecologist with no specific training will produce much lower pregnancy rates.

The use of a laparoscopic approach to salpingostomy needs more evaluation. Selected centres have produced some good results, but overall it appears slightly inferior to those achieved via laparotomy. However, a prospective randomised controlled trial has not been carried out.

A meta-analysis of non-randomised studies investigating the role of magnification for salpingostomy revealed a statistically significant increase in pregnancy rate and decrease in ectopic rate for micro- compared with macrosurgery. A review of 14 series of microsurgical salpingostomy found a cumulative live-birth rate of 21% with an 8% ectopic rate.

Hydrosalpinges

A number of retrospective studies suggest that the presence of hydrosalpinges is associated with decreased implantation and conception rates in patients undergoing IVF-embryo transfer. An increased ectopic rate is certainly recognised. The mechanism is thought to be a combination of embryotoxicity of the hydrosalpingeal fluid combined with poor endometrial receptivity. Uncontrolled studies have found increased implantation rates, pregnancy rates and lower miscarriage rates after removal. The only prospective RCT found no significant difference but was under-powered. It is hoped that the multicentre prospective randomised controlled trial currently in progress in Scandinavia will clarify whether removal prior to IVF will improve pregnancy rates and lessen ectopic rates.

Reversal of sterilisation

Approximately 3% of women will regret being sterilised and a proportion will request reversal. The most common reason is a new relationship. Careful pre-operative counselling can decrease but not eliminate the number of requests. Confirmation of ovulation and semen analysis is mandatory prior to undertaking the procedure. Factors to consider include:

- type of sterilisation performed
- presence of co-existing tubal pathology
- other infertility factors, including the male
- female age.

Sterilisation, particularly with clips but also with Silastic® rings, carries the best prognosis because of minimal tubal damage. Sterilisation by diathermy carries the worst prognosis.

Isthmic-isthmic anastomosis is the most successful. Results are less good when the ampulla is damaged or when there is a wide disparity in the luminal diameter of the two joined segments.

Even in women over 40 years of age, reversal can achieve high intrauterine pregnancy rates, whereas IVF success rates tend to be poor. In general, tubal-factor infertility due to previous sterilisation should be treated by tubal reanastomosis, not IVF. Success rates are related to the experience of the surgeon.

The role of laparoscopic reversal is unclear. High success rates can be achieved using a microsurgical approach. A literature review found a 44–92% overall intrauterine pregnancy rate. Compared with IVF, tubal surgery carries no risk of ovarian hyperstimulation and a lower risk of multiple pregnancy and miscarriage. It also allows for repeated attempts at conception. These, however, are balanced against the risks of major abdominal surgery and an increased ectopic pregnancy rate.

IVF

Most studies considering pregnancy following surgery for proximal and distal tubal disease, tubal reanastamosis and tubal adhesions have found the majority of pregnancies occurring in the first year. Only a few pregnancies occur during the second year and therefore it would be reasonable to discuss IVF with a couple who are not pregnant 12 months after tubal surgery.

IVF OR SURGERY

IVF was first introduced as a method to overcome tubal infertility. It should be considered the first line of treatment for moderate to severe tubal disease and bipolar tubal disease. Previous ectopic pregnancy may also be a contraindication to tubal surgery as recurrence rates are further increased. Overall, it would appear that only 25–50% of women with tubal-factor infertility are suitable for surgery. Before deciding on IVF, the following factors should be considered:

- female age
- severity of tubal disease
- other fertility factors
- the live birth rate per cycle of IVF that can be expected
- risks of ovarian hyperstimulation, multiple pregnancy and, possibly, ovarian cancer
- financial costs.

From 1996–97, women with tubal-factor infertility underwent 11 984 cycles of IVF (35.8% of the total). The live-birth rate was 14.9% compared with 16.7% overall (HFEA 1997).

It is unclear whether the degree of tubal damage present influences pregnancy rates. Maternal age remains overwhelmingly the most important relevant factor.

Another important consideration is number of cycles planned. Despite a putative cumulative pregnancy rate of 60% after three cycles of IVF, most couples in the UK only undergo one or two cycles, thereby reducing their chance of success.

Three economic studies suggest that patient selection and number of IVF cycles are the most important factors in determining the cost effectiveness of surgery and IVF. By narrowing the selection criteria for tubal surgery to women with low-grade tubal disease and women requesting reversal of clip or ring sterilisation, the number of operations can be reduced. Repeated attempts at conception are thus allowed and good live-birth rates can be achieved.

On the other hand, life-table analysis shows a significant increase in the rate of deliveries (72.3% per patient) after three to five cycles of IVF compared with 24% overall following tubal surgery. This is balanced against the risks of ovarian hyperstimulation, multiple pregnancy, and the fact that only 29% of women in the UK have more than one IVF cycle.

Both tubal surgery and IVF should be discussed without bias, bearing in mind that no randomised controlled comparison between the two exists. This is more likely to be achieved in centres offering both microsurgery and IVF services. Prognosis should be tailored to the individual, taking into account local experience and outcomes. The discussion should include comment regarding likely risk factors and financial implications.

KEYPOINTS
- IVF should be discussed if pregnancy has not occurred 12 months after surgery.
- IVF should be considered as the first line of treatment for moderate or severe tubal disease and bipolar tubal disease.
- Maternal age is of greater relevance than the degree of tubal damage in influencing pregnancy rates.

Prevention

Tubal-factor infertility is probably the most preventable type of infertility.

Most abdominal surgery causes adhesions. These can result not only in tubal-factor infertility but also in chronic pelvic pain. Good surgical technique can reduce the risk. This includes:

- use of unpowdered gloves
- minimal tissue handling
- sharp dissection
- constant irrigation
- meticulous haemostasis.

Absorbable adhesion barriers may be considered useful in gynaecological surgery as they significantly decrease the incidence, extent and severity of postoperative adhesions. Their main disadvantage is high cost.

World-wide there has been a change in the prevalence of chlamydial infection. Programmes to decrease the incidence of genital chlamydia infection have not been widely implemented except in Sweden, where screening, contact tracing and free treatment for genital chlamydia have been part of the healthcare system since the 1980s. Declining rates of chlamydial infection, PID and ectopic pregnancy have been attributed to these policies (Egger *et al.* 1998). This contrasts to the situation in the UK and USA where the rate of chlamydial infection and PID continues to rise. The benefits of secondary prevention have been recently demonstrated by a randomised controlled trial which showed that targeted screening could reduce the incidence of PID at one year by 56% (Scholes *et al.* 1996).

Within the UK, the Chief Medical Officer's Expert Advisory Group (1998) has recommended 'action to reduce the prevalence and morbidity associated with chlamydial infection'. Their recommendations include those shown in Table 5.2.

Table 5.2   Recommendations regarding secondary prevention of chlamydial infection of the Chief Medical Officer's Expert Advisory Group (1998)

- Diagnostic testing of such 'at risk' groups as genitourinary medicine clinic (GUM) attendees, women seeking termination of pregnancy, patients with symptoms, and infants with ophthalmia neonatorum and neonatal pneumonitis

- Opportunistic screening of all sexually active women under the age of 25 years and those over the age of 25 years if they have a new sex partner or have had two or more partners in the past 12 months

- Chlamydial screening or antibiotic prophylaxis before uterine instrumentation

---

References

Chief Medical Officer's Expert Advisory Group (1998) *Chlamydia trachomatis – Summary and Conclusions of CMO's Expert Advisory Group.* London: Department of Health

Egger, M., Low, N., Davey Smith, G., Lindblom, B. and Herrmann, B. (1998) Screening for chlamydial infections and the risk of ectopic pregnancy in a county in Sweden: ecological analysis. *BMJ* **316**, 1776–80

Gillett, W.R. and Herbison, G.P. (1989) Tubocornual anastomosis: surgical considerations and coexistent infertility factors in determining the prognosis. *Fertil Steril* **51**, 241–6

HFEA (Human Fertilisation and Embryology Authority) (1997) *Sixth Annual Report.* London: HFEA

Jacobs, L.A., Thie, J., Patton, P.E. and Williams, T.J. (1988) Primary microsurgery for postinflammatory tubal infertility. *Fertil Steril* **50**, 855–9

Penney, G.C., Thompson, M., Norman, J. *et al.* (1998) A randomised comparison of strategies for reducing infective complications of induced abortion. *Br J Obstet Gynaecol* **105**, 599–604

Scholes, D., Stergachis, A., Heidrich, F.E., Andrilla, H., Holmes, K.K. and Stamm, W.E. (1996) Prevention of pelvic inflammatory disease by screening for cervical chlamydia infection. *N Engl J Med* **334**, 1362–6

Thurmond, A.S. (1994) Pregnancies after selective salpingography and tubal recanalisation. *Radiology* **190**, 11–13

Wu, C.H. and Gocial, B. (1988) A pelvic scoring system for infertility surgery. *Int J Fertil* **33**, 341–6

6 Infertility and endometriosis

Introduction

Endometriosis, defined as the presence of viable endometrial tissue outside the uterine cavity, is a common condition affecting 2–3% of women of reproductive age. Many aspects of the pathogenesis of endometriosis are unknown and there is no single theory accounting for its aetiology, which appears to be multifactorial. Today, a composite theory of retrograde menstruation with implantation of endometrial fragments in conjunction with peritoneal factors to stimulate cell growth is the most widely accepted explanation. The sequelae of endometriosis include chronic pelvic pain, severe dysmenorrhoea and infertility. The presence or severity of symptoms does not correspond directly with the extent of the visible disease.

The association with infertility is unclear. Endometriosis is diagnosed in 10–20% of women investigated for infertility compared to 1–5% of women undergoing sterilisation. Despite intense research efforts over the past 50 years, the pathophysiological mechanisms of endometriosis and endometriosis-associated reproductive failure remain incompletely understood. Reduced fecundity in women with moderate and severe endometriosis is readily appreciated due to anatomical alterations associated with pelvic adhesions (Figure 6.1). The effects of minimal and mild endometriosis on fertility are less clear, although the monthly fecundity rate in these women is less than that of the general population (Figure 6.2).

Due to the lack of good quality, prospective, controlled studies and of agreement and consistency in staging, it is uncertain whether the mere presence of endometriosis reduces fertility. It is also possible that an underlying defect, possibly of immunological origin, is responsible for both endometriosis and the infertility in women with endometriosis.

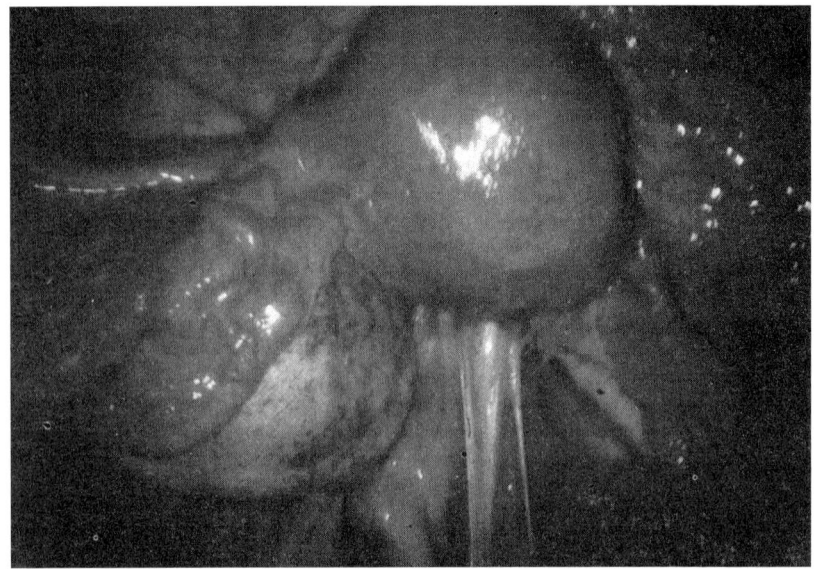

Figure 6.1 Left ovarian endometrioma and peritoneal deposits (reproduced with permission from *An Atlas of Endometriosis*, by RW Shaw, Parthenon Publishing Group)

Mechanisms by which minimal and mild endometriosis may impair fertility

DEFECTIVE FOLLICULOGENESIS

It has been suggested that, in women with endometriosis, ovulation may be disturbed by an abnormality of the follicular growth rate and total growth period, or that altered intra-ovarian mechanisms might be responsible for abnormal follicular recruitment, growth and selection in endometriosis patients. However, it has been shown that there is no significant difference in daily peripheral endocrinology, folliculogenesis, endogenous LH surge and growth of endometrial thickness among women with or without endometriosis.

DISORDERS OF OVULATION

Luteinised unruptured follicle syndrome is the condition where, following normal follicular growth and oestrogen secretion, the follicle fails to rupture and release the oocyte and this is followed by luteinisation of the granulosa cells. Laparoscopic examination of women during the luteal phase and serial ultrasound scanning have been used to investigate whether this occurs more often in patients with endometriosis, without

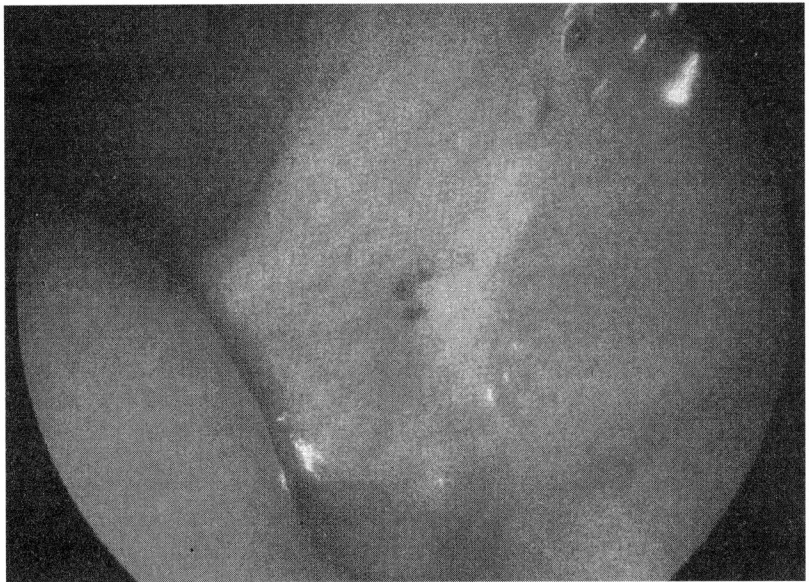

Figure 6.2 Mild endometriosis (reproduced with permission from *An Atlas of Endometriosis*, by RW Shaw, Parthenon Publishing Group)

any conclusive evidence being found for this hypothesis. It has also been suggested that anovulation is more common in infertile women with endometriosis, but this has never been confirmed.

HYPERPROLACTINAEMIA

Hyperprolactinaemia has been reported in patients with mild endometriosis varying from 11% to 36%. It has been suggested that women with endometriosis demonstrate a significant increase in the prolactin response to thyroid-releasing hormone (TRH). However, in further studies this increase was found to be confined to patients with severe endometriosis. The mechanism by which women with endometriosis exhibit significant prolactinaemia following LHRH/TRH test is unclear. The administration of bromocriptine as a therapeutic measure has been tried, but available data suggest that it is ineffective.

LUTEAL PHASE DEFICIENCY

The diagnosis of luteal phase deficiency is based upon either:

- the duration of the luteal phase
- an aberrant basal body-temperature chart and endometrial biopsy
- a low level of progesterone production.

It was initially suggested that women with endometriosis demonstrated decreased progesterone production during the luteal phase. However, studies have shown that luteal progesterone production in such women is normal, based on single and multiple progesterone estimations. It is therefore reasonable to conclude that a luteal phase defect is not the mechanism by which the majority of women with endometriosis are rendered infertile.

AUTO-IMMUNITY

It has been suggested that sensitisation to endometrial antigens could occur as a part of the inflammatory response to the retrograde menstrual debris: the resultant auto-antibodies could thus interfere with the process of fertilisation and possibly implantation. An increase in the number of T cells, B cells and the ratio of CD4/CD8 lymphocytes in patients with endometriosis in both peritoneal fluid and peripheral blood has also been reported. The methods used in many of these studies were non-specific and some of the earlier findings were later refuted by further studies.

KEYPOINTS
- Due to the lack of controlled studies and of agreement on the consistency of staging, it is uncertain whether the presence of endometriosis reduces fertility.
- The majority of studies are inconclusive regarding the possible mechanisms by which minimal and mild endometriosis may impair fertility.

Peritoneal environment

Endometriosis can now be regarded as a local inflammatory process in the pelvis. The local environment of peritoneal fluid surrounding the endometrial implant is immunologically dynamic and links the reproductive and immune systems. The fallopian tubes and ovaries are bathed in peritoneal fluid. Spermatozoa are exposed to peritoneal fluid factors in the fallopian tube before and during fertilisation, as are oocytes and embryos.

The volume of peritoneal fluid in patients with endometriosis may be increased, but this appears to be of little clinical importance and correlates poorly with infertility. However, peritoneal fluid components may negatively affect the reproductive environment. This may be associated with the increased concentration of macrophages that exist in the presence of endometriosis. It is becoming evident that cytokines, released by macrophages, play an important role in reproduction at various levels, including gamete function, fertilisation and embryo development, implantation and postimplantation survival of the conceptus. Overall, there appears to be enough evidence to suggest that the peritoneal environment in women with endometriosis is relatively hostile to the process of conception.

KEYPOINTS
- Endometriosis is more frequently diagnosed among infertile women than in fertile women.
- In advanced endometriosis adhesion formation and tubal damage can directly affect fertility.
- The aetiology of infertility in minimal and mild endometriosis is not well understood.

Treatment of endometriosis and reproductive outcome

The management of endometriosis remains contentious. There are many reports in the literature on therapeutic options for endometriosis, but well-designed studies supporting the efficacy and effectiveness of these interventions are not always available. This is particularly true for women with minimal and mild disease, in whom no clear causal association can be defined. The options for treatment of endometriosis-associated infertility include:

- no treatment
- medical treatment with or without surgery
- surgical treatment by laparoscopy or laparotomy.

The published studies have many methodological problems, including heterogeneity in clinical characteristics, such as stage of disease and the presence of other infertility factors, in addition to small sample sizes and variable duration of follow-up.

MEDICAL TREATMENT
Pharmacological agents used for the medical treatment of endometriosis include:

- continuous combined oral contraceptive preparations
- progestogens alone
- danazol

- gestrinone
- GnRH-agonists.

In the treatment of endometriosis-associated infertility, the highest quality data available demonstrate no benefit from ovulation suppression when compared to placebo or no treatment, whatever the stage of the disease. Three systematic reviews with meta-analysis, all using slightly different methodologies, have consistently shown that there is no significant difference in crude pregnancy rates between medical treatment and no treatment in endometriosis. In the cohort and prospective studies included in the most recent meta-analysis (Adamson and Pasta 1994), there was no evidence to suggest that medical treatment of endometriosis improved fertility. Therefore, medical treatment causing ovulation suppression is not appropriate for endometriosis-related infertility. Larger trials of this approach do not appear to be warranted on the basis of available data.

SURGICAL TREATMENT

In moderate and severe endometriosis, comparisons of surgical treatments with non-surgical alternatives show that surgery is generally superior, when comparing pregnancy rates. There is, however, no evidence of a difference between laparoscopic and open (laparotomy) approaches.

It is less clear whether surgery is superior to no treatment in minimal and mild disease. Laparotomy for the treatment of minimal or mild disease would generally be regarded as inappropriate. Data from nine studies comparing laparoscopic surgery with no treatment in minimal and mild endometriosis show an increased relative risk of pregnancy of 1.6 (95% CI 1.4–1.8), suggesting a benefit from laparoscopic resection or ablation. Within the studies included, the only well-designed randomised trial was by Marcoux *et al.* (1997). In the trial, 341 infertile women with minimal and mild endometriosis were randomised to either diagnostic laparoscopy alone or surgical treatment of the endometriosis with destruction and removal of all visible endometriotic implants and lysis of adhesions. The results suggested that laparoscopic surgery increased the cumulative probability of a pregnancy by 73% in the first 36 weeks after the procedure. This suggests a benefit from resection or ablation of endometriosis to one in eight women with minimal or mild disease undergoing such a procedure. However, it must be emphasised that there are some concerns regarding the design of the trial. The patients were not blinded regarding the group to which they were randomised, 14% of women had lysis of adhesions as well as destruction of endometriosis and a small number of patients also underwent co-interventions such as ovulation induction, IVF/IUI, progestogens, cyst excision and contraception. However, for the moment, the available evidence, for all its shortcomings, does suggest a benefit from surgical intervention in this group of patients. It is clear, however, that there is a need for further controlled prospective studies which present their results for different stages of endometriosis using comparable classification systems.

ADJUVANT TREATMENT

The evidence suggests that in the management of endometriosis-associated infertility, the addition of post-operative medical treatment does not improve pregnancy rates compared to surgery alone. This is true whether the surgery is laparoscopy or laparotomy. From this evidence and the evidence that medical treatment alone does not improve pregnancy rates compared with no treatment, it is clear that medical treatment has no role in the management of endometriosis-associated infertility.

There is still the possibility that presurgical medical treatment could be a beneficial adjunct. The theoretical advantages of medical treatment before surgery are reduced inflammation and vascularisation and shrinkage of implants. However, the quality of evidence supporting the use of medical treatment before conservative surgery for endometriosis is poor, and no recommendations could be made based on the results of the published studies.

KEYPOINTS
- Evidence suggests that medical treatment has no role in the management of endometriosis-associated infertility.
- Surgery is generally superior to non-surgical alternatives in moderate and severe endometriosis.
- Subfertile women also benefit from surgical ablation of minimal and mild endometriosis.

Assisted reproduction in endometriosis-related infertility

Pelvic endometriosis refractory to medical or surgical therapy currently accounts for between 7% and 35% of patients undergoing IVF procedures. All stages of endometriosis have increasingly been viewed as suitable indications for assisted reproduction treatment. However, it is not known whether IVF or gamete intrafallopian transfer (GIFT) is better than medical or surgical treatment for endometriosis associated infertility. Following the advent of assisted reproduction, more patients with endometriosis failing to conceive with conventional therapy have been treated with one or the other of these techniques. The timing of assisted reproduction is dependent upon the severity of the disease and any previous therapy, as well as other factors, such as female age and duration of infertility.

There are no direct comparisons of relevance but some evidence suggests that IVF or GIFT may be better than conventional treatment for women with endometriosis, whatever the stage of disease (Table 6.1). As far as the success of IVF/GIFT treatment is concerned, large national registers have repeatedly reported similar pregnancy rates for women with endometriosis in comparison with other categories. The presence or the degree of endometriosis does not appear to affect the fertilisation or embryo cleavage rates, and more particularly the live birth rates following treatment.

Evidence on the use of IUI in the treatment of endometriosis-associated infertility suggests that ovarian hyperstimulation with IUI is more effective than either no treatment or IUI alone in women with minimal or mild disease.

Table 6.1   Use of assisted reproduction in endometriosis-related infertility

Severity of endometriosis	Treatment
Minimal or mild	IVF or GIFT treatment after more than two years of surgical or expectant management IUI with ovarian hyperstimulation may be an effective alternative to IVF (used for at least 3 cycles)
Moderate or severe	IVF should be considered one year after unsuccessful surgery IVF may be considered in preference to surgery depending on the clinical situation
Severe, with mechanical blockage and where surgical therapy is inappropriate	IVF should be expedited

> *KEYPOINTS*
> - The timing of assisted reproduction is dependent on the severity of the disease and any previous therapy, as well as other factors, such as female age and duration of infertility.
> - IVF or GIFT may be better than conventional treatment for women with endometriosis, whatever the stage of disease.
> - In cases of moderate and severe endometriosis, assisted reproductive techniques should be considered, as an alternative to or following unsuccessful surgery.
> - In cases of minimal or mild disease IVF or IUI with ovarian stimulation may be considered after more than two years of surgical or expectant management.

Conclusion

The nature of the relationship between endometriosis and infertility remains unresolved. It is unclear whether endometriosis causes infertility or whether there is an underlying defect that causes both infertility and endometriosis. However, there seems to be enough evidence to suggest that drugs suppressing ovulation are of no benefit in infertile women with endometriosis and their use only delays the likelihood of a spontaneous pregnancy or more effective treatments such as IVF.

References

Adamson, G.D. and Pasta, D.J. (1994) Surgical treatment of endometriosis-associated infertility: meta-analysis compared with survival analysis. *Am J Obstet Gynecol* **171**, 1488–504

Marcoux, S., Maheux, R. and Berube, S. (1997) Laparoscopic surgery in infertile women with minimal or mild endometriosis. *N Engl J Med* **337**, 217–22

7 Unexplained infertility

Introduction

Unexplained infertility is the term used to describe the situation in which a couple whose routine investigations of semen analysis, tubal patency and assessment of ovulation yield normal results. Intrinsic differences within populations and variations in investigation protocols have led to a wide range in the reported prevalence of unexplained infertility. Values range from 5.8% to 58%, but most clinics now report incidences of 20–30%. The distinction has been made between the diagnosis of unexplained infertility in a couple as opposed to that in an individual. A typical example of the latter is the female partner of an azoospermic male who fails to conceive after repeated attempts of donor insemination despite having a normal pelvis and biochemical evidence of ovulation.

The clinical approach to unexplained infertility has undergone a major shift in emphasis in the last decade. Traditionally, the aim has been to identify possible (mainly female) causes for the condition in the hope of devising appropriate therapy. In the absence of a definite diagnosis, couples were subjected to a variety of empirical treatments. In recent years, with the availability of assisted reproduction, many of the old diagnostic exercises are no longer seen to be crucial to the management of the condition. Instead, there is increasing reliance on evidence-based medicine and awareness of the need to limit the adverse effects of any treatment.

This chapter briefly considers the relevance of some of the putative causes of unexplained infertility before assessing common treatment strategies.

Possible causes of unexplained infertility

Failure of routine tests to detect any obvious contributory factors has led clinicians to speculate about numerous subtle causes for unexplained infertility. Although many areas remain of interest to researchers, their practical relevance has been diminished by the growing role of assisted reproduction (Table 7.1).

Table 7.1 Possible aetiologies of unexplained infertility

Possible cause	Comments
Luteal-phase deficiency	Lack of consensus about both diagnosis and treatment of this condition have challenged its clinical relevance in recent years.
Luteinised unruptured follicle syndrome	Clinical usefulness is compromised by the lack of uniformity of ultrasonic criteria for defining this syndrome.
Hyperprolactinaemia	Evidence linking subtle endocrine abnormalities to unexplained infertility is tenuous.
Endometriosis	It is uncertain whether the mere presence of endometriosis reduces fertility.
Subclinical pregnancy loss	The prevalence of this condition in unexplained fertility has been shown to be no different from that in the general population.
Anatomical abnormalities	These are of little relevance in the causation of unexplained infertility.
Occult infection	The role of infection *per se* in the genesis of unexplained infertility is unproven.
Sperm dysfunction	It is likely that cases of unexplained infertility are associated with subtle disorders of sperm function as well as sperm-mucus and sperm-oocyte interaction which can only be exposed by IVF.
Immunological causes	A clear link between the presence of antisperm antibodies and unexplained infertility is yet to be established.
Psychological factors	Proof of a direct correlation between objectively defined stress levels and unexplained infertility is unavailable.

The concept of luteal-phase deficiency as a cause of unexplained infertility remains a controversial topic. It is presumed to be due to defects in folliculogenesis and luteal function. Potential mechanisms include:

- Abnormalities of gonadotrophin secretion
- Intrinsic ovarian defects
- Defects of endometrial steroid receptors
- Abnormalities of luteal rescue.

While delays in histological maturation of the endometrium have been documented as proof of the existence of this condition, its effect on fertility is unclear. Lack of consensus about both diagnosis and treatment of this condition have challenged its clinical relevance in recent years.

LUTEINISED UNRUPTURED FOLLICLE SYNDROME

Failure of the leading follicle to rupture in the presence of biochemical evidence of ovulation has been linked to unexplained infertility. Following the LH peak, serial ultrasound scans have identified failure of the dormant follicle to shrink in a group of women with low serum progesterone levels. Its clinical usefulness is compromised by the lack of uniformity of ultrasonic criteria for defining this syndrome (see also Chapter 6).

HYPERPROLACTINAEMIA

The role of prolactin in ovulatory disorders remains uncertain. High levels of prolactin may be associated with deficient luteal function. Both transient elevations of prolactin in the luteal phase and absence of the midcycle elevation of prolactin have been demonstrated in women with unexplained infertility. However, prolactin-lowering agents such as bromocriptine have been ineffective in treating women with unexplained infertility.

Although it is difficult to identify specific hormonal abnormalities in women with unexplained infertility, intensive monitoring can reveal subtle changes suggestive of diminished ovarian reserve. The limitations of screening for mild ovarian dysfunction are generally accepted. Evidence linking other subtle endocrine abnormalities to unexplained infertility is tenuous and there is little justification for empirical hormonal treatment.

ENDOMETRIOSIS

Although strictly speaking a separate condition, mild endometriosis without gross distortion of pelvic anatomy has traditionally been linked to unexplained infertility. The possible effects of minimal endometriosis and the implications of its treatment are considered in Chapter 6.

SUBCLINICAL PREGNANCY LOSS

Once thought to be an important factor in unexplained infertility, the prevalence of this condition, which is dependent on the sensitivities of the screening tests used, has been shown to be no different from that in the general population.

ANATOMICAL ABNORMALITIES

Tubocornual polyps and other subtle anatomical aberrations are of little relevance in the causation of unexplained infertility and their treatment seems to have minimal effect.

OCCULT INFECTION

Impaired tubal function due to previous infection with *Chlamydia trachomatis* has been cited as a possible aetiology for unexplained infertility. Although chlamydial infection is clearly important in the context of tubal disease, the role of infection *per se* in the genesis of unexplained infertility is unproven. Currently there is no evidence to support the empirical use of antibiotics (see also Chapter 5).

SPERM DYSFUNCTION

Conventional semen analysis represents a crude method of assessing male fertility, particularly as it cannot evaluate the functional capacity of spermatozoa. However, it is likely that some cases of unexplained infertility are associated with subtle disorders of sperm function as well as sperm-mucus and sperm-oocyte interaction, which can only be exposed by IVF. Cellular defects of sperm may relate to the generation of abnormal amounts of free oxygen radicals, which could affect the stability of the sperm membrane. Such sperm may be functionally incompetent despite possessing normal laboratory parameters. Though sophisticated tests of sperm function remain useful research tools, access to assisted reproduction and the current role of IVF as a test of gamete function limit their role in current management of unexplained infertility (see also Chapter 3).

IMMUNOLOGICAL CAUSES

Serological tests have identified the presence of antisperm antibodies capable of inhibiting fertilisation, although a clear link between the presence of these antibodies and unexplained infertility is yet to be established. Antiphospholipid antibodies, including antibodies to any one of five to seven phospholipid antigens, have been linked with infertility. As assays for antiphospholipid antibodies other than anticardiolipin are not standardised, this is a difficult association to prove.

PSYCHOLOGICAL FACTORS

Though infertility is undoubtedly stressful, proof of a direct correlation between objectively defined stress levels and unexplained infertility is not available. In addition, no controlled studies exist that show a link between reduction of stress and enhanced fertility in this group.

KEYPOINTS
- Unexplained infertility is a diagnosis of exclusion in the presence of normal semen parameters, evidence of ovulation and tubal patency.
- The practical relevance of research into subtle causes for unexplained infertility has been diminished by the growing role of assisted reproduction.

Diagnosis

Investigation of the infertile couple is discussed in Chapter 2. It is worth noting that for complete evaluation of the pelvis a diagnostic laparoscopy with dye transit is the procedure of choice. Where basic tests for ovulation, semen parameters and tubal patency are all normal and the pelvis is unremarkable, a diagnosis by exclusion is made. Unexplained infertility has traditionally been associated with a plethora of tests, few of which contribute significantly to either the choice or the success of treatment. Thus, in routine cases, it is not practical or cost effective to screen for each of the many causes discussed above. In the light of current evidence it is difficult to justify the use of tests like endometrial biopsy, serial progesterone levels and ovarian scans in an attempt to diagnose luteal-phase deficiency. Sperm function tests and tests for antisperm antibodies are also not recommended for routine use. Much debate still surrounds the use of the postcoital test. Although vigorously supported by its proponents, its clinical usefulness has always been questionable. Current evidence from a recent randomised trial failed to show any benefit of this test in enhancing pregnancy rates – a view endorsed by the recent RCOG evidence-based guidelines. Other investigations that have yet to be shown to be clinically useful include screening for antiphospholipid antibodies, hysteroscopy and ultrasound of the endometrium (RCOG 1998).

Management

From the outset, it must be appreciated that the management of unexplained infertility has certain unique features:

1   In the absence of a certain diagnosis, any form of treatment is, by definition, empirical.

2 Treatment, even with relatively invasive assisted reproduction techniques, produces only fairly modest pregnancy rates.

3 In couples with unexplained infertility there always exists a chance of a spontaneous pregnancy and this must be taken into account when treatment is considered.

This background pregnancy rate is strongly affected by the duration of infertility (Figure 7.1). A period of three years of unexplained infertility is generally accepted as the minimum duration before considering active intervention. In couples who have been trying for less than three years, the likelihood of spontaneous pregnancy over the next two years is 46% as compared with 27% in those with a longer duration of infertility (Collins *et al.* 1995). Apart from duration of infertility, the female partner's age and previous pregnancy history have a major effect on spontaneous conception rates as well as treatment outcome (Table 1.3).

Models for estimating the chances of conception for individual couples have been devised to aid better insight into planning treatment. As a general rule, in women under 35 years of age, conservative treatment for up to three years should be considered, since spontaneous conception rates only start to decline significantly after this period (Collins and Rowe 1989). Successful communication with the couple is vital at

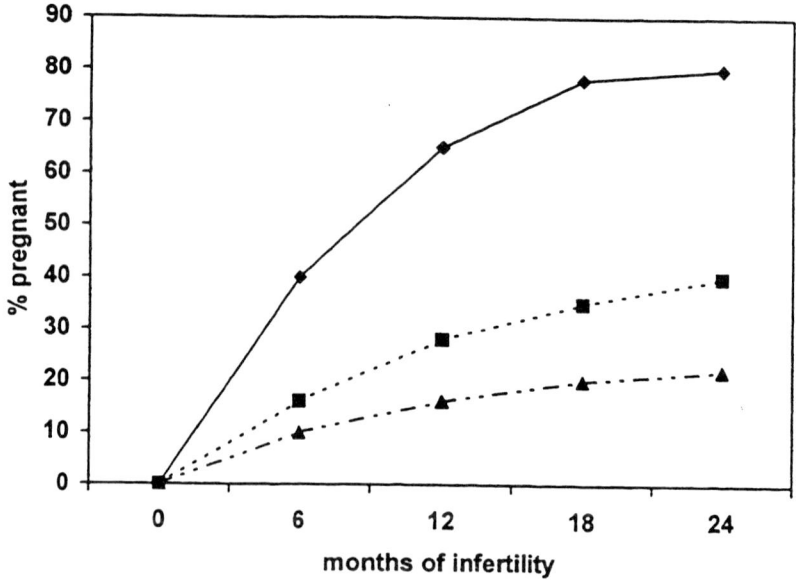

Figure 7.1 Prognosis in unexplained infertility: effect of duration of infertility; – – ▲ – – = one year; -■- = three to five years; –– = over five years

this point and the importance of detailed discussion and written information sheets cannot be overstated. Many couples feel frustrated by the apparent refusal to accede to their request for early treatment and they need careful counselling. Once the expectant role is abandoned, it is important to identify the treatment of choice and formulate a clear plan of future management. When a number of options are available it may be appropriate to start with the one that is least invasive. Management should be evidence-based and in keeping with the wishes of the couple. Financial constraints can introduce a further layer of complexity into the decision making process.

The effectiveness of some of the commonly used forms of treatment is discussed below.

EMPIRICAL CLOMIPHENE

Clomiphene citrate has been shown to increase the number of follicles produced per cycle, thus increasing the odds of a fertilised embryo reaching the uterine cavity (see Chapter 4). While undoubtedly effective in anovulatory infertility, its use in unexplained infertility is still open to debate. The current evidence comes from a number of randomised trials with insufficient power to make any conclusions about the effect of clomiphene on pregnancy rates. Inevitably, any comments regarding effectiveness must be based on the results of systematic reviews of clinically heterogeneous trials. A recent meta-analysis has demonstrated a clinically and statistically significant benefit following the use of clomiphene in unexplained infertility (Hughes *et al*. 1998a). The combined odds ratio (OR) for clinical pregnancy per patient was 2.37 (95% CI 1.43–3.94). Another systematic review by the same author (Hughes 1997), this time using a different methodology, failed to confirm the independent effect of clomiphene on pregnancy rates.

Since the publication of these studies, a randomised trial has shown that clomiphene is ineffective in ovulatory women. When these latest results are added to those derived from the first meta-analysis, the combined odds ratio falls to 1.4 with confidence levels crossing unity, confirming that clomiphene results in little or no benefit. The large number of relatively small trials inevitably means that the present conclusions are likely to be affected by the outcome of future studies.

Traditionally, clomiphene has been viewed as a relatively innocuous drug and its empirical use is preferred by many to the more invasive assisted-reproduction techniques. Concerns about clomiphene-induced multiple pregnancy and an inability at present to rule out a potential link with ovarian cancer underline the need to weigh the risk-benefit ratio carefully. Current evidence suggests that treatment with clomiphene results in little or no benefit in unexplained infertility (RCOG 1998). Until further evidence is available, it is difficult to justify its use outside the context of a randomised trial.

DANAZOL AND BROMOCRIPTINE

Other drugs used for the treatment of unexplained infertility include danazol and bromocriptine. The rationale for their use is the putative association of hyperprolactinaemia and minimal endometriosis with unexplained infertility. Unlike the debate about clomiphene, the verdict here is quite clear. Recent meta-analyses of trials involving both these agents have attested to their total lack of effectiveness in this context (Hughes *et al.* 1998b,c).

SUPEROVULATION AND INTRAUTERINE INSEMINATION

Superovulation with IUI has been a recognised treatment for unexplained infertility for a number of years. Though this approach is less invasive than IVF, significant risks of ovarian stimulation and multiple pregnancy remain. Current evidence regarding this treatment comes from a meta-analysis of eight randomised controlled trials comparing FSH/IUI with FSH/timed intercourse in unexplained infertility (Hughes 1997). This suggests a significant improvement in pregnancy rates associated with IUI following ovulation induction (OR 2.37; 95% CI 1.43–3.90). A second systematic review assessed the independent effects of FSH, clomiphene and IUI across all diagnostic categories of infertility. Analysis of 22 trials indicated that the OR for pregnancy associated with FSH use was 2.35 (95% CI 1.87–2.94), and for IUI the odds ratio was 2.82 (95% CI 2.18–3.66). A synthesis of the above data provides the best available evidence, indicating that the likelihood of pregnancy is approximately two-fold higher with FSH and nearly three-fold higher with IUI. The inference is that combination of the two has a summative effect increasing the odds further, perhaps by a factor of five. Clinically this implies that superovulation with IUI should be offered to couples with unexplained infertility prior to embarking on IVF. Compared with superovulation with IUI, superovulation alone has the dual disadvantages of lower pregnancy rates while maintaining comparable risks of hyperstimulation and multiple pregnancy. IUI without superovulation has seldom been tried for unexplained infertility. Although theoretically an attractive proposition, because it offers a three-fold increase in pregnancy rates without the complications and cost associated with gonadotrophins, there is a paucity of clinical data to support this form of treatment and further evidence is needed before it can be recommended.

GIFT

In cases where the pelvis has been shown to be normal, it seems reasonable to perform GIFT, that is, replace the gametes within the tubes rather than subject them to *in vitro* culture. This obviates the need for a sophisticated embryology laboratory. While the outcome of treatment with GIFT on the whole has been encouraging, results from two randomised trials suggest that the outcome following ovarian stimulation with IUI may be similar to that achieved by GIFT. A third trial, however, suggests that GIFT is more effective. Given the more invasive nature of GIFT, it seems reasonable to offer a limited number of superovulation/IUI cycles before progressing to GIFT or IVF. IVF has been shown to be just as effective as GIFT but may be preferred on the basis of its ability to provide important diagnostic information regarding fertilisation without subjecting that patient to the risks of general anaesthesia and laparoscopy. Despite its undoubted efficacy in treating couples with unexplained infertility, current evidence suggests that in centres capable of offering IVF, this should be the treatment of choice (RCOG 1998).

IVF

Treatment of unexplained infertility that is prolonged or refractory to other forms of treatment is best undertaken by IVF. Though empirical, this technique has the undisputed merit of being able to circumvent most of the hypothetical causes of unexplained infertility including ovulation dysfunction, cervical factors and sperm-egg interaction. Initially devised as a treatment for tubal-factor infertility, IVF has been shown to be as effective in other types of infertility. Women under 35 years of age with three to four years of unexplained infertility unresolved by superovulation/IUI are best treated by IVF, which has a diagnostic role in identifying any problems with fertilisation. In older women, despite the relatively poorer prognosis, IVF should be considered after a shorter duration of infertility.

It has been suggested that, in cases of unexplained infertility, unsuspected problems with sperm-oocyte interaction may result in poor fertilisation rates. These couples may need intracytoplasmic sperm injection (ICSI) in future cycles. Though concern about failed fertilisation has prompted some clinicians to consider ICSI to be the definitive treatment of unexplained infertility, evidence from clinical trials does not support this view. Preliminary results from a randomised controlled trial comparing the two types of treatment have failed to show either improved fertilisation rates or pregnancy rates with ICSI.

COMPARISON OF TREATMENT REGIMES FOR UNEXPLAINED FERTILITY	
Treatment	*Comments*
Clomiphene citrate	Confers little or no benefit Concerns regarding clomiphene-induced multiple pregnancy and a potential link with ovarian cancer
Danazol and bromocriptine	Not effective
Superovulation/IUI	May increase odds of pregnancy by a factor of five Should be offered to all couples before embarking on IVF treatment
Superovulation alone	Likelihood of pregnancy twice as high Lower pregnancy rates than combined treatment Comparable risks of hyperstimulation and multiple pregnancy
IUI alone	Three-fold increase in pregnancy rates without the complications and cost associated with gonadotrophins More evidence is needed before treatment can be recommended
GIFT	Similar or potentially more effective treatment than superovulation/IUI More invasive
IVF	Ability to provide important diagnostic information regarding fertilisation Less invasive than GIFT Treatment of choice if infertility unresolved by superovulation/IUI Able to circumvent most of the hypothetical causes of unexplained infertility

Conclusion

Unexplained infertility continues to present a diagnostic and therapeutic challenge. Advances in assisted reproduction have improved outcome

> **KEYPOINTS**
> - The main factors affecting outcome are duration of infertility, female age and parity.
> - Expectant treatment is recommended unless the duration of infertility is more than three years or the female partner is more than 35 years of age.
> - Effective treatments include superovulation with intrauterine insemination and IVF. The role of empirical clomiphene is debatable.

for many couples and simplified our management of the condition but many questions still remain unanswered.

There is little justification for investigations other than biochemical tests for ovulation, semen analysis and pelvic assessment by laparoscopy.

The outcome of unexplained infertility depends on the duration of infertility, female age and parity. While treatment must be tailored to the individual couple, active intervention is not recommended unless the duration of infertility is more than three years or the female partner is more than 35 years of age.

Effective treatments include superovulation with IUI and IVF. The role of empirical clomiphene is debatable.

References

Collins, J.A. and Rowe, T.C. (1989) Age of the female partner is a prognostic factor in prolonged unexplained infertility. *Fertil Steril* **52**, 15–20

Collins, J.A., Burrows, E.A. and Wilan, A.R. (1995) The prognosis for live birth among untreated infertile couples. *Fertil Steril* **64**, 22–8

Hughes, E., Collins, J. and Vanderkerckhove, P. (1998a) Clomiphene citrate vs placebo or no treatment in unexplained infertility (Cochrane Review). *The Cochrane Library,* Issue 2. Oxford: Update Software

Hughes, E., Tiffen, G. and Vanderkerckhove, P. (1998b) Danazol vs placebo in unexplained infertility (Cochrane Review). *The Cochrane Library,* Issue 2. Oxford: Update Software

Hughes, E., Collins, J. and Vanderkerckhove, P. (1998c) Bromocriptine with placebo in women with unexplained infertility (Cochrane Review). *The Cochrane Library,* Issue 2. Oxford: Update Software

Hughes, E.G. (1997) The effectiveness of ovulation induction and intrauterine insemination in the treatment of unexplained infertility: a meta-analysis. *Hum Reprod* **12**, 1865–72

RCOG (1998) *The Management of Infertility in Secondary Care.* London: RCOG Press (Evidence-based clinical guidelines No. 3)

8 Assisted conception techniques

Introduction

The term 'assisted conception' is used to describe a number of techniques employed to treat infertility. One of these techniques may be the final option for many couples with intractable pathology, failed primary treatment or unexplained infertility. Techniques employed include:

- IVF
- GIFT
- zygote intrafallopian transfer (ZIFT)
- tubal embryo stage transfer (TEST)
- intrauterine insemination (IUI)
- donor insemination (DI)
- egg donation
- intracytoplasmic sperm injection (ICSI)
- embryo cryopreservation
- surrogacy.

There have been marked improvements in these methods in the past few years, particularly in the field of male factor infertility and micromanipulation. For the last ten years, success rates – presented as live-birth rate per treatment cycle – seems to have reached a plateau for IVF at 14–15%, whereas in micromanipulation rates rose from 4% to 22% (HFEA 1998). The procedures, their nomenclature, indications, technical basis and results are summarised in Table 8.1.

In practice, the time to choose assisted conception methods is when the chance of pregnancy is otherwise down to only 1–2% or less in each cycle and the cumulative chance amounting to less than 25% during the course of two years' exposure to natural conception.

The outcome of treatment is determined particularly by:

- the age of the woman
- any previous pregnancy
- initial FSH levels

Table 8.1 Techniques used in assisted reproduction

Technique	Principle	Major indications	Outcome (pregnancy per cycle)
IVF	Oocyte retrieval under ultrasound guidance Insemination, embryo culture and transcervical replacement, mostly between pronucleate and eight-cell stage	Tubal disease Pelvic adhesions impeding ovum pick-up Sperm antibodies Selected semen abnormalities	15–20%
GIFT	Oocyte retrieval and replacement with sperm into tubal ampulla at laparoscopy	Infertility of any cause where tubes are normal and semen quality is adequate Unexplained infertility	20–25%
ICSI	IVF in which a single sperm is injected into the cytoplasm to allow fertilisation	Severe oligozoospermia in the male or successive failed fertilisation	20%
OD	Oocyte retrieval under ultrasound guidance and transcervical replacement of embryos into the recipient's endometrial cavity	Absent or non-functioning ovaries or carriers of a serious genetic disorder	20–30%
IUI	Use of prepared partner's semen for insemination usually following ovulation induction or superovulation	Unexplained infertility	2–10%
DI	Use of prepared donor semen for insemination	Azoospermia or oligozoospermia in the male partner	10%

- duration of infertility
- the number of eggs or embryos available for replacement at the end of the treatment.

This chapter will focus on those methods which involve bringing oocytes and sperm together. They almost invariably take advantage of multiple ovulation and always require selective preparation of the sperm in culture medium before delivery to the oocytes.

In vitro fertilisation

IVF is suitable for women with tubal disease, ovulatory disorders, endometriosis, in couples with unexplained infertility of longer than three years duration and in the presence of oligoasthenozoospermia. There are several steps in the IVF procedure and technical variations inherent in the treatment can have an important impact on success.

OVARIAN STIMULATION

Superovulation is invariably employed, not only because success depends on the number of embryos or oocytes transferred, but also to facilitate the control and the timing of oocyte collection. The aim of any regimen for stimulating multiple follicular development for assisted conception is to obtain as many follicles as possible from which good quality eggs can be recovered. These eggs should be able to be fertilised and produce embryos which are 'developmentally competent' – that is, they are capable of forming a viable pregnancy. In addition, the regimen should have a low complication rate and not result in hyperstimulation.

Pituitary desensitisation using a GnRH analogue is often employed prior to and during ovarian stimulation. The desensitisation brings great practical advantages by blocking the endogenous LH surge, which reduces the necessity of cancelling cycles. Ovarian stimulation, for many years, has been achieved by hMG extracted from the urine of menopausal women. However, even purified urinary FSH contains significant contamination with urinary proteins. More recently, recombinant gonadotrophins (r-FSH and r-LH) have become available, making possible the use of gonadotrophins which are virtually devoid of exogenous proteins. Superovulation is described in Chapter 4.

OOCYTE RETRIEVAL

The ultrasound-guided oocyte retrieval is usually performed under light sedation and analgesia; combinations of benzodiazepines, midazolam and opiates are given intravenously or intramuscularly, with appropriate monitoring both during and after the procedure. More recently, the use of patient-controlled analgesia during oocyte retrieval has produced satisfactory results. The patient is awake and often accompanied by her partner. Collected oocytes can be shown to the couple on a closed-circuit video monitor attached to the embryologist's microscope. It is important that the patient is counselled carefully prior to the procedure as the oocyte retrieval can occasionally be painful and anxious patients may require heavy sedation or even general anaesthesia.

The procedure itself takes 15–20 minutes. A single or double lumen needle, attached to an electronic pump, enables rapid aspiration of every follicle and also allows 'flushing' of the follicle in the case of double lumen needles. It is important to recognise that follicles may not always contain an oocyte of adequate quality. Furthermore, oocytes obtained following repeated follicular flushing fertilise less well and may produce poor-quality embryos.

SPERM-OOCYTE MIXTURES

After oocyte retrieval, sperm is washed and prepared and might be enhanced by reagents that improve fertilisation. Insemination is usually performed one to six hours after oocyte retrieval with 50 000–20 0000 motile spermatozoa being placed with each oocyte. Following an incubation period of 16–18 hours the oocytes are examined to ensure that normal fertilisation has occurred, as defined by the presence of two pronuclei. Multiple pronuclei indicate polyspermic fertilisation or digyny (i.e. failure to extrude the second polar body) and such oocytes are not suitable for transfer. Suitable embryos are kept in incubation until they are transferred into the uterine cavity or cryopreserved.

MICRO-ASSISTED FERTILISATION

ICSI is a relatively new technique which involves the direct injection of a single sperm through the outer membranes of the oocyte to reach the cytoplasm (Figure 8.1). A variation of this technique (called subzonal sperm injection, SUZI) involves the injection of the sperm between the zona pellucida and vitelline membrane. However, only ICSI offers a significant benefit over standard mixing of oocytes with washed sperm and other methods are no longer used. The main indication for ICSI is failure of fertilisation, which is a common problem in male-factor infertility (see Chapter 3).

This treatment has revolutionised the management of couples suffering from male-factor infertility, who previously would have to resort to donor insemination as the only option with a realistic chance of producing a

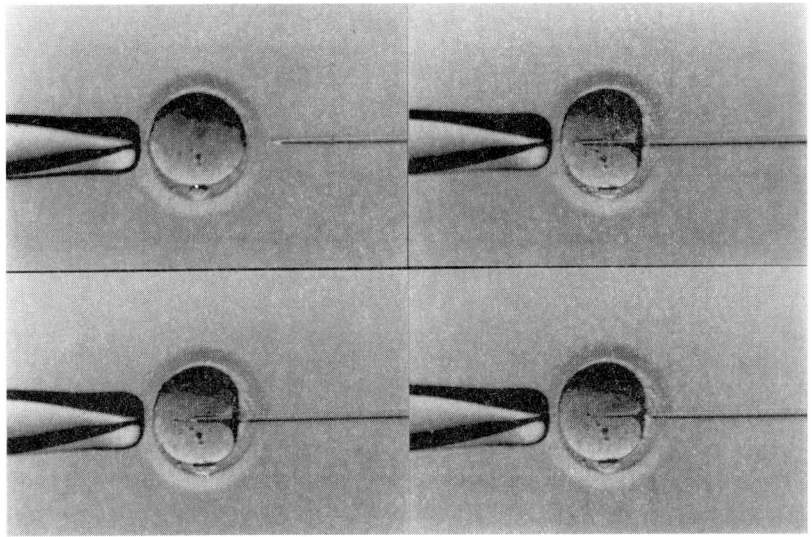

Figure 8.1 Injection of a single spermatozoa into an oocyte

pregnancy. Success rates have risen significantly during the course of the last ten years and have recently reached 21% live-birth rate per cycle of treatment (HFEA 1998). Success with micromanipulation seems higher than with IVF, although this may not be the case when corrected for female factors. Micromanipulation of the embryo can also be performed in the form of 'assisted hatching' which may improve implantation rates for patients with previous IVF failures.

Safety concerns have been expressed regarding the use of micro-manipulation techniques, especially of ICSI, as we have limited knowledge about the natural selection of the spermatozoa for fertilisation. The safety of micro-assisted fertilisation remains to be established, but the data on children born to date as a result of ICSI treatment are reassuring with respect to congenital abnormalities.

EMBRYO TRANSFER

In IVF cycles, the optimal time for embryo transfer is between 48 and 72 hours following the oocyte collection (at the four- to eight-cell stage). Research is under way to see if prolonged *in vitro* culture to the blastocyst stage (day five) will improve the ability to select better quality pre-embryos for transfer. In the UK, it is prohibited to replace more than three embryos under the Human Fertilisation and Embryology Act 1990. However, because of the risk of multiple pregnancy, it is recommended that all couples give serious consideration to having a maximum of two embryos replaced, with the cryopreservation of the extra embryos. This policy results in fewer multiple pregnancies and reduces the risk of a triplet pregnancy, while not reducing significantly the cumulative 'take-home baby' rate.

SUCCESS RATES

A clinical pregnancy is defined by a rising level of hCG combined with ultrasound visualisation of a gestational sac. A live birth is defined as any birth event in which at least one baby is born and survives for more than a month. While there are variations between centres providing IVF treatment, it is clear that well-established centres consistently achieve pregnancy rates of around 25% and live-birth rates of around 20% per commenced cycle in women under 40 years of age and men with normal sperm function (HFEA 1998).

Individual success rates, being unrelated to the cause of infertility, can vary greatly according to age, duration of infertility, previous pregnancy and previous unsuccessful IVF attempts. The woman's age is a well-known factor influencing the outcome of fertility treatment. Results decline sharply after the age of 40 years, the decline beginning around the age of 36 years. Live-birth rates are highest in the age group 25–30 years; 17% at age 30 years and virtually zero by 45 years of age (Table 8.2). Women who have achieved a previous pregnancy have a significantly higher live-birth rate than women who have had no previous pregnancies. This effect is stronger for previous live births, previous IVF pregnancies having the strongest effect. A history of a previous IVF pregnancy is associated with a live-birth rate of 23.2%, compared with 12.5% for a woman with no previous pregnancy.

Table 8.2   Live birth rates by age of woman (Source: HFEA Annual Report 1998)

Age (years)	Live birth rate (IVF)	Micromanipulation using own eggs (%)
< 27	18	27
30	20	28
35	14	22
40	10	12
45	1	3

CRYOPRESERVATION OF GAMETES AND EMBRYOS

Cryopreservation of donor sperm or patient's sperm prior to chemotherapy provides an opportunity for the sperm to be used for assisted fertilisation at a later date. Sperm is frozen in 7.5% glycerol at –196°C in liquid nitrogen and there is apparently no biological time limit to cryopreservation. Cryopreservation of oocytes has not been very successful to date. It might be that cryopreservation of ovarian tissue followed by autografting or *in vitro* culture of follicles will provide a better chance of viable oocytes for women about to undergo chemotherapy or radiotherapy.

In embryo cryopreservation, embryos are stored in liquid nitrogen at –196°C, usually at the pronuclear or early cleavage stages. Embryo survival is in the region of 70%. Thawed embryos are transferred two to three days after ovulation in carefully monitored natural cycles or three days after the commencement of progesterone therapy in artificial cycles in which down-regulation has been performed with a GnRH analogue and oral oestradiol given until the endometrium has developed adequately. The HFEA permits embryo storage for up to ten years, although there is no evidence that deterioration occurs beyond this time.

KEY POINTS
- Superovulation is invariably employed.
- The advent of ICSI treatment has revolutionised the management of couples suffering from male-factor infertility.
- It is recommended that all couples should consider having a maximum of two embryos replaced.
- Women who have achieved a previous IVF pregnancy have the highest live-birth rate.

Gamete intrafallopian transfer

GIFT is the procedure where gametes (the female oocyte and the male sperm) are transferred surgically into the fallopian tube at the time of oocyte collection. Fertilisation, therefore, takes place within the fallopian tube. The ovulation induction is exactly the same as in IVF but the oocytes can be collected laparoscopically. Only women with healthy, and not just patent, fallopian tubes are suitable for GIFT and their partners must have a normal semen analysis as 50 000–20 0000 prepared sperm are placed in the fallopian tube for each oocyte. In the UK, a maximum of three oocytes per treatment cycle is usually transferred and any extra oocytes are inseminated for subsequent freezing and storage.

A drawback of GIFT is not knowing whether the oocytes which have been replaced into the tubes are fertilised or not and the procedure requires a general anaesthetic and laparoscopy. These problems may be offset by the apparently higher success rates with GIFT treatment compared with IVF, regardless of the woman's age and regardless of whether or not male-factor infertility is present. Results from the USA, where GIFT is more commonly employed than in the UK, suggest a 24% delivery rate per oocyte retrieval, compared with 15% following IVF.

Variations of the routine GIFT technique are ZIFT and TEST:

1   In ZIFT, following IVF, transfer into the fallopian tube is carried out laparoscopically at either the pronucleate or single cell (zygote) stage
2   In TEST the transfer is at the cleaving embryo stage.

KEY POINTS
- Ovulation induction is the same as in IVF but the oocytes can be collected laparoscopically.
- Only women with healthy fallopian tubes are suitable for GIFT and their partners must have a normal semen analysis.

Intrauterine insemination

Intrauterine insemination (IUI) is a relatively less invasive technique defined as direct transfer of motile spermatozoa into the uterine cavity, after sperm preparation and concentration in a small volume of medium. Indications for IUI include:

- cervical mucus problems
- coital or ejaculatory disorders
- the presence of sperm antibodies
- mild male-factor infertility
- unexplained infertility
- conventional donor insemination.

Ovarian stimulation is often used to induce multiple ovulation. However, depending on the indication for IUI, it is possible to employ the technique in carefully monitored natural, ovulatory cycles. If ovarian stimulation is employed, clomiphene citrate, tamoxifen or hMG can be used for this purpose. Pituitary down-regulation is usually not employed and the ovarian response is monitored by ultrasound examinations.

Ultrasound examinations are carried out between the 10th and 12th day of the cycle and if a response of at least one follicle (but not more than three) greater than 16 mm in diameter is confirmed, then a single dose of hCG or r-LH is administered. Following LH administration, insemination is carried out 24–48 hours later. If four or more mature follicles are detected on the ultrasound examination most units would not carry out the insemination, in order to reduce the risk of a multiple pregnancy, and would recommend barrier contraception. An alternative to IUI is direct intraperitoneal insemination (IPI, DIPI) of the washed sperm via the posterior vaginal fornix, although this is not common practice.

> *KEY POINTS*
> - IUI is a relatively less invasive technique.
> - Ovarian stimulation is often used.
> - If four or more follicles are detected on ultrasound examination, insemination would probably not be carried out.

Donor insemination

The main indication for treatment by donor insemination is azoospermia (absence of spermatozoa) or oligozoospermia (reduced numbers of spermatozoa) in the male partner (see Chapter 3). The use of donor semen may also be considered:

- following vasectomy
- following failed vasovasotomy
- following ejaculatory dysfunction
- following chemotherapy or radiotherapy
- to prevent the transmission of a genetic disorder
- (rarely) for severe rhesus isoimmunisation with a homozygous rhesus-positive male partner.

Donor recruitment is performed in accordance with the British Andrology Society (1993) guidelines. The selection and screening of sperm donors has to be scrupulous, not only to ensure that the frozen sperm has a good chance of achieving a pregnancy but also to prevent the transmission of diseases to the recipient. Donors should be between the ages of 18 and 55 years (HFEA 1990) and are screened for:

- cystic fibrosis
- gonorrhoea
- *Chlamydia trachomatis*
- human immunodeficiency virus (HIV)
- hepatitis
- syphilis
- cytomegalovirus (CMV).

In the UK, the HFEA requires sperm to be cryopreserved for at least six months in order for the donor screening tests to be completed and the HIV test repeated.

All couples who undergo DI have to accept independent counselling, both as an essential part of the treatment and as a prerequisite of the HFEA. They need to understand how donors are selected and screened and the limitations of accurate matching. The counsellor should also describe the law with respect to the legal position of the child and the parents and also the rules governing confidentiality and anonymity.

Ovarian stimulation is only indicated for anovulatory cycles. In ovulatory cycles, insemination is timed to coincide with ovulation. This is best determined by daily monitoring of serum LH levels or using home ovulation predictor kits. The live-birth rate for DI has increased steadily over the last five years, and has almost doubled since 1992. According to the latest figures, following DI, the live-birth rate per cycle of treatment is around 10% for stimulated and 9% for unstimulated cycles (HFEA 1998). Cumulative pregnancy rates of 40–50% after six and 70–80% after 12 inseminations, in women under the age of 35 years are reported. Live-birth rates for DI decrease with woman's age, increasingly so after the age of 35 years.

KEY POINTS

- In the UK, the HFEA requires sperm to be cryopreserved for at least six months in order for donor screening tests to be completed.
- All couples who undergo DI must accept independent counselling.
- Ovarian stimulation is only indicated for anovulatory cycles.

Ovum donation

Ovum donation is required when the woman is a known carrier of a serious genetic disorder, where her ovaries are absent, non-functioning or are unlikely to respond to ovulation induction. Oocytes are obtained from healthy volunteers younger than 35 years of age who are screened for:

- infection (syphilis, gonorrhoea, hepatitis and HIV)
- cystic fibrosis.

As with sperm donation, extensive independent counselling is required for the recipient couple and the donor. Donor anonymity is preferred and leads to fewer long-term problems. Donors undergo ovarian stimulation as in IVF cycles. The collected oocytes are inseminated with the recipient's partner's sperm and the resulting embryos are transferred into the recipient's uterus. It is necessary to provide the recipient with hormone replacement therapy (HRT), usually with increasing doses of oral oestrogens and the addition of progesterone three days before embryo transfer, which continues for at least another 10–14 days. Recipients who have a spontaneous menstrual cycle require pituitary desensitisation before commencing the hormone regimen, while amenorrhoeic women with ovarian failure do not. Interestingly, it is the latter group who appear to have better results, possibly because the HRT regimen is not imposed on a pre-existing cycle. Close synchrony is required between the recipient's cycle and the donor's IVF cycle if fresh embryos are to be transferred.

Pregnancy rates are essentially dependent on the age of the donor. However, with the increasing age of the recipient, there is also a slight decline in success rates, possibly due to endometrial ageing or acquisition of gynaecological problems, such as fibroids.

KEY POINTS
- Independent counselling is required for both the recipient couple and the donor.
- Donor anonymity is preferred and leads to fewer long-term problems.
- Donors undergo ovarian stimulation, as in IVF cycles.
- Amenorrhoeic women with ovarian failure appear to have better results than those with a spontaneous menstrual cycle.

Surrogacy

Surrogacy is a legal form of assisted reproduction technology applicable only to a small number of couples. The primary medical indication for use of surrogacy is the inability of a woman to provide the genetic and/or the gestational component for childbearing.

Complete surrogacy:	Sperm from the partner of the infertile woman is used to inseminate the surrogate mother, who will carry the pregnancy and give the resulting child over to the couple. The couple then adopts the child.
Partial surrogacy:	The woman has intact ovaries but is unable to gestate due to an absent or severely malformed uterus. The couple can create an embryo *in vitro*, then have it transferred to the uterus of the surrogate

---

The ethical aspects of surrogacy are considerable and it is essential that the surrogate host and her partner as well as the couple receive independent counselling before embarking upon treatment.

HUMAN FERTILISATION AND EMBRYOLOGY AUTHORITY

- The regulation of infertility treatment in the UK is undertaken by the Human Fertilisation and Embryology Authority (HFEA), which was established following the Human Fertilisation and Embryology Act 1990.

- The first statutory body of its type in the world, the HFEA's creation reflected public and professional concern for the potential future of human embryo research and infertility treatments, and a widespread desire for statutory regulation of this ethically highly sensitive area.

- The HFEA's principal tasks are to license and monitor those clinics which carry out IVF, DI and human embryo research.

- The HFEA also regulates the storage of gametes (sperm and eggs) and embryos.

Conclusion

The introduction of assisted reproduction techniques has provided effective treatment for infertile men and women and stimulated continuing research in the field of reproduction. The requirement for assisted conception is seldom absolute infertility, but is mostly some degree of subfertility. The choice of treatment therefore depends on a balance of factors, including the duration of infertility and the woman's age.

GIFT appears to have an advantage in success rates over IVF for women with healthy tubes and men with normal sperm, but this treatment involves laparoscopy and general anaesthesia.

The safety of micro-assisted fertilisation remains to be established although initial reports are encouraging in this respect. The rational development and deployment of IVF and the techniques of micro-assisted fertilisation holds at least the promise of a solution for many couples. For clinicians, the challenge is to deploy these new techniques sensibly and effectively.

References

British Andrology Society (1993) British Andrology Society guidelines for the screening of semen donors for donor insemination. *Hum Reprod* **8**, 1521–3

HFEA (UK Human Fertilisation and Embryology Authority) (1990) *Code of Practice*. London: HMSO

HFEA (UK Human Fertilisation and Embryology Authority) (1998) *Seventh Annual Report*. London: HMSO

Glossary

ART	assisted reproductive technique
BAS	British Andrology Society
CASA	computer-assisted sperm analysis
CBAVD	congenital bilateral absence of the vas deferens
CFTR	cystic fibrosis transmembrane conductance regulator
cGMP	cyclic guanosine monophosphate
CMV	cytomegalovirus
DSS	diagnostic selective salpingography
DIPI	direct intraperitoneal insemination
DI	donor insemination
DTO	distal tubal occlusion
E$_2$	oestradiol
FSH	follicle-stimulating hormone
GIFT	gamete intrafallopian transfer
GMP	guanosine monophosphate
GnRH	gonadotrophin-releasing hormone
hCG	human chorionic gonadotrophin
HEPT	zona free hamster egg penetration test
HIV	human immunodeficiency virus
hMG	human menopausal gonadotrophin
HRT	hormone replacement therapy
IBT	immunobead test
ICSI	intracytoplasmic sperm injection
IHH	idiopathic hypogonadotrophic hypogonadism
IUCD	intrauterine contraceptive device
IUI	intrauterine insemination
IVF	*in vitro* fertilisation
LH	luteinising hormone
LHRH	luteinising hormone-releasing hormone
LPD	luteal phase deficiency
LUF	luteinised unruptured follicle
MAR	mixed agglutinin test

OD	ovum donation
OHSS	ovarian hyperstimulation syndrome
PCOS	polycystic ovary syndrome
PCT	postcoital test
PIF	prolactin inhibitory factor
PTO	proximal tubal obstruction
STD	sexually transmitted diseases
SUZI	subzonal sperm injection
TC	tubal catheterisation
TEST	tubal embryo stage transfer
TFI	tubal factor infertility
TRH	thyrotropic-releasing hormone
TSH	thyroid-stimulating hormone
ZBT	zona binding test
ZIFT	zygote intrafallopian transfer

Recommended reading

Baker, H.W.G. and Keogh, E.H. (1994) 'Update on male infertility' in: J. Bonnar (Ed.) *Recent Advances in Obstetrics and Gynaecology*, pp. 109–25. Edinburgh: Churchill Livingstone

Royal College of Obstetricians and Gynaecologists (1998) *The Initial Investigation and Management of the Infertile Couple*. London: RCOG Press (Evidence-based Clinical Guidelines No. 2)

Royal College of Obstetricians and Gynaecologists (1998) *The Management of Infertility in Secondary Care*. London: RCOG Press (Evidence-based Clinical Guidelines No. 3)

Shaw, R.W. (1995) *Endometriosis, Current Understanding and Management*. Oxford: Blackwell Science

Templeton, A.A. and Drife, J. (1992) *Infertility. Proceedings of the Royal College of Obstetricians Study Group*. London: RCOG Press

Templeton, A.A., Cooke, I. and O'Brien, P.M.S. (Eds) (1998) *Evidence-based Fertility Treatment*. London: RCOG Press

Index